It Only Takes a Second

Preventing Childhood Traumatic Injuries

It Only Takes a Second

Preventing Childhood Traumatic Injuries

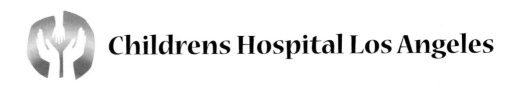

Childrens Hospital Los Angeles

DELMAR
™
THOMSON LEARNING

Australia Canada Mexico Singapore Spain United Kingdom United States

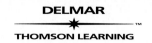

DELMAR

™

THOMSON LEARNING

It Only Takes a Second: Preventing Childhood Traumatic Injuries
Childrens Hospital Los Angeles

Health Care Publishing Director:
William Brottmiller

Product Development Manager:
Marion S. Waldman

Project Development Editor:
Jill Rembetski

Editorial Assistant:
Robin Irons

Executive Marketing Manager:
Dawn F. Gerrain

Channel Manager:
Gretta Oliver

Executive Production Manager:
Karen Leet

Production Editor:
James Zayicek

Production Editor:
Mary Colleen Liburdi

Cover Design:
William Finnerty

Cover Image:
Evan Richardson
Fortissimo Photography

For permission to use material from this text or product,
contact us by
Tel   (800) 730-2214
Fax   (800) 730-2215
www.thomsonrights.com

Library of Congress Cataloging-in-Publication Data

It only takes a second : preventing childhood traumatic
injuries / Childrens Hospital of Los Angeles.
      p. cm.
   ISBN 0-7668-2386-5
   1. Children's accidents—Prevention. 2. Children—
Wounds and injuries—Prevention. 3. Children—Health
and hygiene. I. Childrens Hospital of Los Angeles.
   RD93.5C4 I88 2000
   617.1'0083—dc21

                                        00-064525

The medical leadership of Childrens Hospital Los Angeles
is dedicated to the welfare of all children and to injury
prevention and anticipatory guidance.

Childrens Hospital Los Angeles
4650 Sunset Boulevard
Los Angeles, CA 90027
(323) 669-4531

contents

foreword

Did you know that today's leading health issue for children isn't cancer, heart defects, or any other disease? It's trauma from preventable injuries. You may be surprised to learn, as I was, that injuries kill more of our children than all diseases combined.

That's why I am pleased to be able to draw much needed attention to this problem. And to let you know there are many ways we can help prevent or minimize injuries to our children. They're here in this book.

As a concerned parent, I am especially pleased this vital information comes from someone we can trust: physicians and trauma experts at Childrens Hospital Los Angeles, one of our nation's finest pediatric hospitals and a leader in treating and preventing injuries to infants, children, and teenagers.

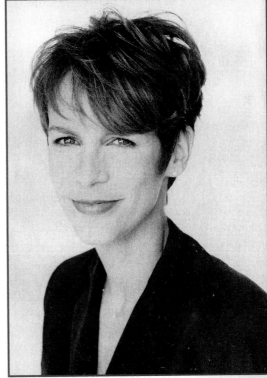

PHOTO BY ANDREW ECCLES

Whether you are a parent, grandparent, family member, or guardian, you'll find tools within these pages that could help you save the life of a child.

We never think an injury will happen to us or someone we love—and then it does. Our children are on the move, exploring the world around them. They're riding in cars, racing bikes, swimming, skating, playing soccer, and crossing traffic. They're at home in the city or the country—in the kitchen, the bath-room, the backyard, watching television. All places where injuries occur.

The good news is that we can do something about this. This book will explode myths about where and how children get injured, and teach you ways to prevent injuries and reduce their severity. It may even change your thinking about accidents. Because what you may consider accidents—injuries that just happen because kids will be kids—are usually preventable. Most important, by preventing these incidents in the first place, we can protect our children from pain and trauma or even worse.

I'm grateful to have this information close at hand for my family. I urge you to read and use this book. Make your child's world safer today.

For our children,
Jamie Lee Curtis

acknowledgments

There are so many people to thank. First, we would like to thank Pamela M. Griffith, Trauma Program Manager at Childrens Hospital Los Angeles for her direction; Robin Moore, Manager of Creative Services at Childrens Hospital Los Angeles for her creative leadership; Candace Pearson for her story editing; the entire Patient and Family Care Services staff at Childrens Hospital Los Angeles for their translation services and authorship regarding pediatric outcomes and Lessons Learned; Yolanda Davalos-Gonzalez, Patricia Gutierrez, and Marlen Bugarin for their assistance in working with our bilingual families; Janet Dotson for her insight with our celebrity families; and Rosa Hernandez, Mimi Yero, Jackie Rosenberg, Judy Branca, Josefina Austriaco, and Ivy Baker for their data collection efforts.

Childrens Hospital Los Angeles is also eternally grateful to all the families that participated and offered their time, understanding, and experiences. You are Childrens Hospital Los Angeles.

Finally, we would like to thank all the contributing experts, most especially Dr. Kathryn D. Anderson, Surgeon-in-Chief at Childrens Hospital Los Angeles, for her support, and Steven Stylianos, MD. We also thank the Children's National Medical Center in Washington, D.C., for their contribution. Last but not least, Margaret Mary Kozik Richardson, Director of Corporate Relations and Technology Transfer at Childrens Hospital Los Angeles, for her project guidance and making this happen.

introduction

Traumatic injuries represent the most significant threat to the health of children in the United States and are the leading cause of death after the first year of life [1]. Injured children account for one-half to two-thirds of all pediatric ambulance runs nationwide, one-fourth to one-half of all pediatric emergency department visits, and one-sixth of all pediatric intensive care unit admissions [2]. More than 20,000 children and young adults will die this year as a result of injury; and for every child that dies, another 40 will require hospitalization and 1,000 more will be evaluated in emergency departments. The cost injuries exact is staggering—approaching nearly $16 billion [3]. Moreover, 50,000 children and adolescents will sustain some degree of permanent disability, the majority victims of brain injury. Morbidity after the initial convalescence remains the most significant determinant of long-term care and quality of life. While expectations may be that children will eventually "outgrow" residual impairments, studies have shown that children may actually "grow into" additional deficits as developmental demands in language and reasoning increase.

These statistics should scare any parent. As former Surgeon General and current chairman of the National Safe Kids Campaign, Dr. C. Everett Koop suggests, we should be outraged by any laissez-faire attitude toward childhood injury, the cause of more pediatric deaths than all other causes combined. Collectively, as parents, grandparents, educators, and caretakers, we can take steps to significantly reduce the devastating effects of this preventable disease by using the information and resources provided in this book [4].

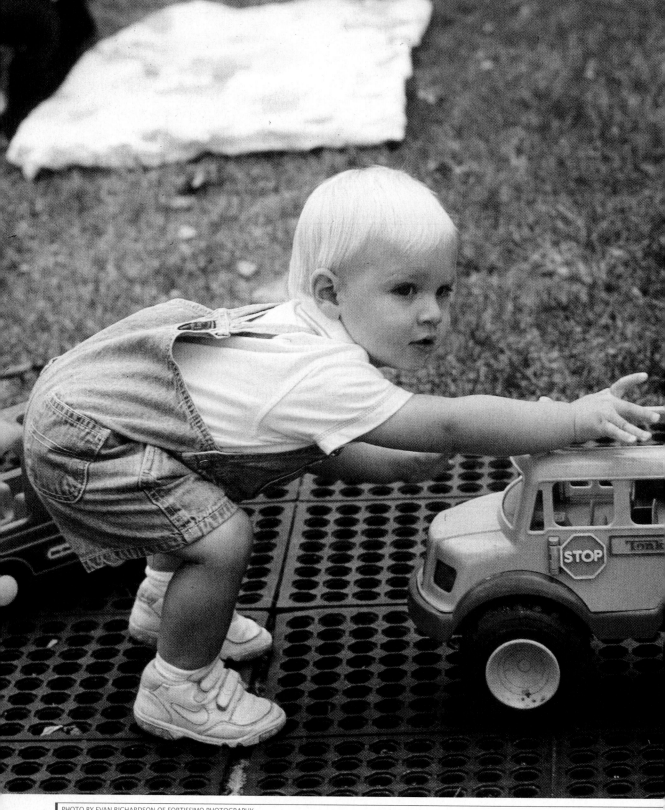

home

The stories you are about to read are all real. The stories feature real parents talking about the lessons they have learned. Please carefully read each story and then take time to implement the safety tips suggested by both the parents and experts. Remember that it could save your child's life.

Nearly 3,000 children under the age of five died in 1998 due to unintentional home injuries [5]. This number should startle and sadden you because your home is the one place over which you have the most control as a parent. Improving the safety of your home includes more than just a one-time childproofing. It is an ongoing activity and includes choosing the appropriate toys, beds, and clothes, following yard and outdoor safety precautions, and being ever vigilant. Parents should also take the time to include fire, tornado, or earthquake safety plans in their overall approach. If a child is injured it is also your responsibility as a parent, grandparent, or caretaker to know what to do. Take cardiopulmonary resuscitation (CPR) classes and stay updated. Know how to perform the Heimlich maneuver if someone is choking and keep a basic first aid kit with you at all times. Finally, be aware of any product recalls. Information on product recalls is available from the U.S. Consumer Product Safety Commission.

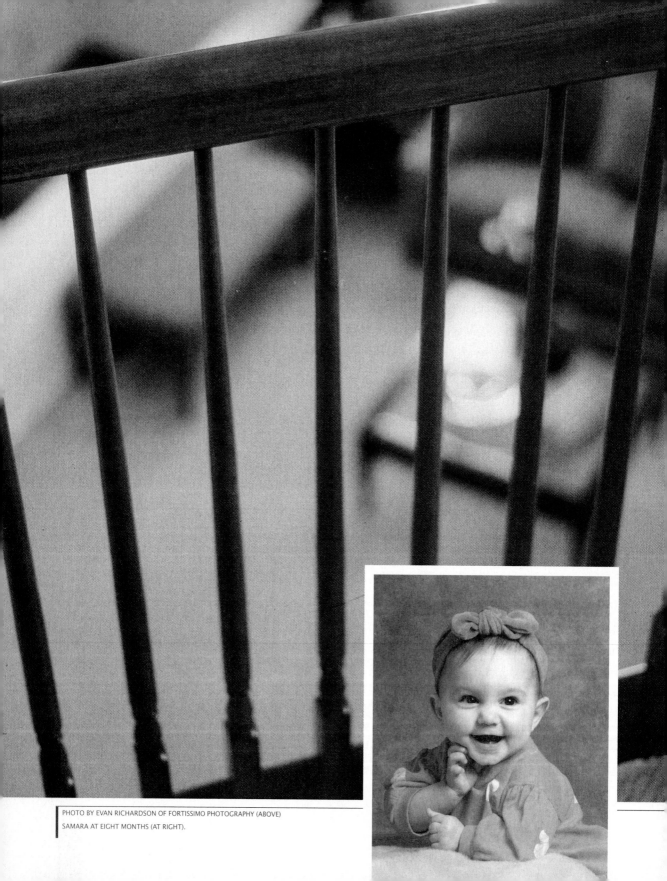

PHOTO BY EVAN RICHARDSON OF FORTISSIMO PHOTOGRAPHY (ABOVE)
SAMARA AT EIGHT MONTHS (AT RIGHT).

It Takes Only One Second

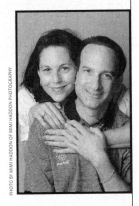

Our daughter, Samara, was only thirteen months old. She was beautiful, petite, and just starting her life. I had just finished speaking with my husband over the telephone about dinner plans and we had decided to order take-out. I closed the baby gate at the top of the stairs and went downstairs to get the restaurant's telephone number. As I was walking back up the stairs, I saw Samara falling. Somehow she squeezed between the railings on the stairwell. Samara was rushed to Childrens Hospital Los Angeles but all the heroic efforts of Samara's doctors could not save her life. The slats of the railing Samara fell through were 4½ inches apart and we were led to believe met the current city building codes, however, that did not save Samara's life.

As parents, we must remember that just because something meets code does not necessarily mean that it is safe for our children. Rather, we must never develop a false sense of security and must actively prevent injuries to our children by "babyproofing" our home and being ever vigilant. Life-altering injuries can take place in seconds, therefore, as parents we can never assume that our child is safe.

—*Barbara and Manuel Weiskopf*

A CLOSER LOOK

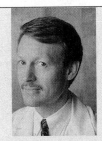

DR. DONALD SHAUL, *Attending Pediatric Surgeon, Division of Pediatric Surgery, Childrens Hospital Los Angeles, and Associate Professor of Surgery, Keck School of Medicine, University of Southern California*

Head injuries are a leading cause of death in children. The key to decreasing the incidence of pediatric brain injuries lies in prevention. Young children must be constantly supervised and safety meshing should be used on all stair and balcony railings.

Causes of Similar Injuries

- Stairs
- Windows
- Beds and cribs
- Countertops
- Wet floors
- Loose rugs
- Stools and other furniture that children can climb

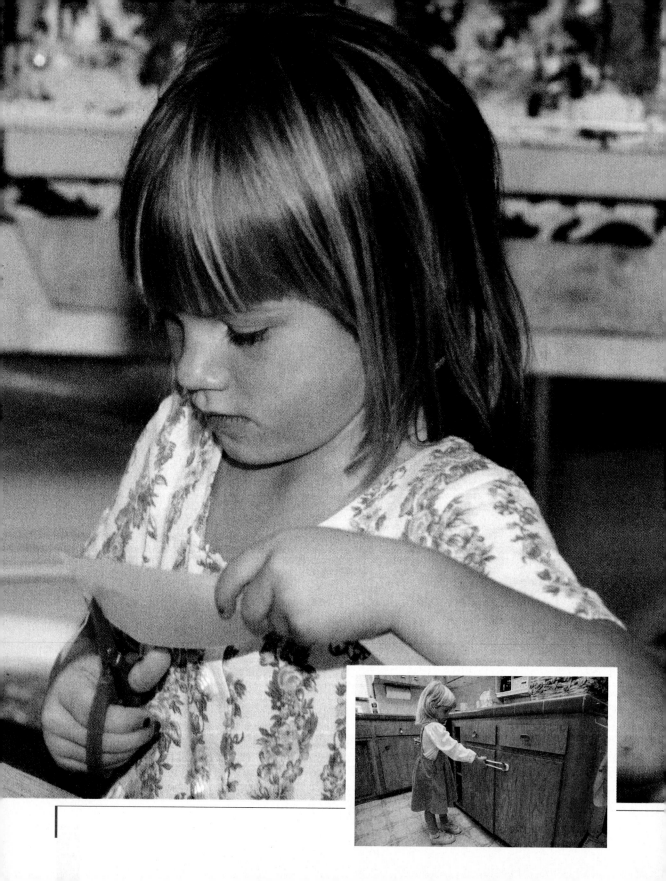

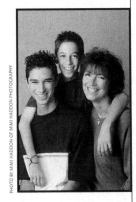

The Pain of Lingering Guilt

The day my son Evan's eye was punctured with a knife stands out as the worst day of my life. Evan, his older brother Justin, and I came home from a holiday shopping trip. Both boys were excited about assembling a model of a space monster we had purchased. I was in another room putting away gifts when I heard seven-year-old Evan screaming. "My eye, my eye!" At first, all I could see was blood seeping through Evan's fingers. When I gently pulled his fingers from his face, his entire eye was filled with blood. We raced to the emergency room of the nearest hospital. On the way, I learned what had happened. When Justin was unable to find scissors to open the package, he decided to use a knife. As Justin entered the living room with the knife, Evan literally ran into the blade.

Luckily, Evan received great care and his vision remains 20/20, after two serious operations and annual visits to the surgeon. The lingering guilt of his brother is not so easily repaired. I have reminded my sons to use the right tools—safely. But the real lesson for every parent is that guilt, regret, and fear can take much more time than physical injuries to heal.

—*Sherry Nolan-Hirschberg*

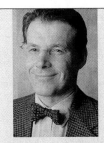

A CLOSER LOOK

Dr. Mark Borchert, *Division Head, Division of Ophthalmology, Childrens Hospital Los Angeles, and Associate Professor of Ophthalmology and Neurology, Keck School of Medicine, University of Southern California*

It is impossible to eliminate the many hundreds of such potentially dangerous objects from a child's environment. Nonetheless, certain precautions can be taken to reduce the risk of eye injuries to children. It goes without saying that children should not be permitted to play or run with sticks or sharp objects. Other hazards may be less obvious. Wire coat hangers should be switched to plastic. Tables should have rounded rather than sharp corners. Drawers and cabinets should be latched closed to keep toddlers from potentially dangerous objects, as well as to prevent them from running into the corner of a drawer inadvertently left open. Additional information is available from the Protective Eyewear Certification Council (PECC), c/o Paul F. Vinger, M.D., 297 Heath's Bridge Road, Concord, MA 01742; or on-line at www.protecteyes.org.

Causes of Similar Injuries

- Toothbrush
- Scissors
- Sticks

Install Safeguards

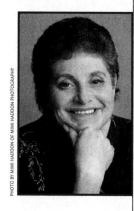

When my daughter, Tanya, was about two years old, she took a tumble in our house and hit her face on a table—a fairly common occurrence for toddlers, but in this case it resulted in stitches and a visit to the hospital. At the time, very few safety items were available for the home. Today, a simple bumper guard around our table would have softened the blow to Tanya's face and nose. Ignorance isn't "bliss" when it comes to safety.

Especially now as I look forward to being a grandparent, I would strongly encourage grandparents to become familiar with safety equipment and install all appropriate items. Then stay updated on equipment as it is introduced. Grandparents must make a special effort to childproof their homes to protect visiting grandchildren. This will reduce the anxiety of the visit for everyone—and definitely decrease the severity of any injury.

—Dr. Arleen Forsheit

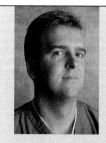

A CLOSER LOOK

Dr. Richard J. Cartie, *Pediatric Critical Care Fellow, Division of Critical Care Medicine, Childrens Hospital Los Angeles*

Injuries to toddlers most often take place at home. When children learn to walk and interact with their environment, everyday objects can become deadly. Solid furniture with corners or edges should be out of traffic areas, where access can be limited. Fireplace hearths should be padded for safety, as should kitchen island corners. Efforts should also be made to use electrical outlet covers, properly store electrical cords, and safety gates.

Causes of Similar Injuries

- Coffee table
- Kitchen island
- Kitchen table
- Banister
- Fireplace hearth

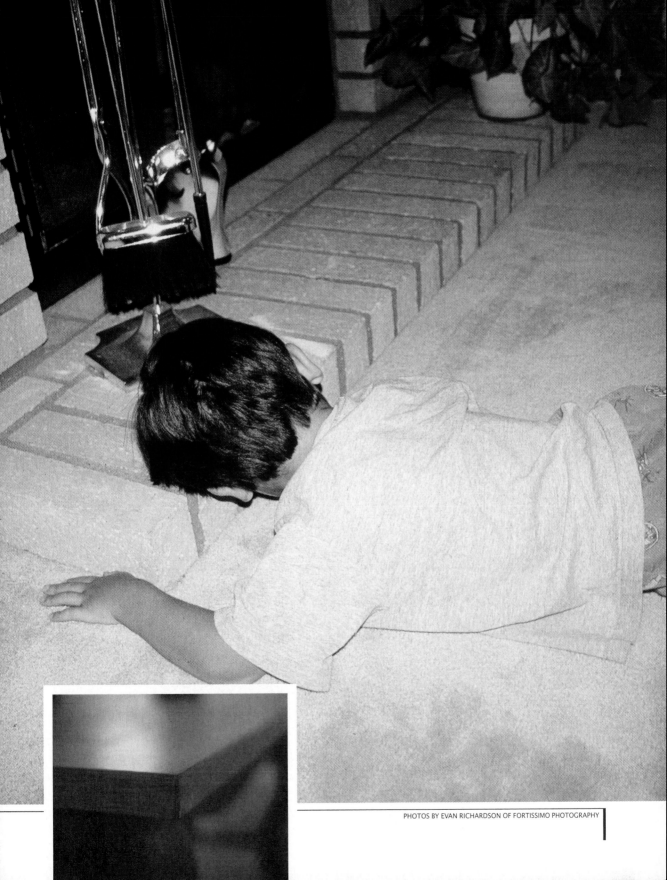

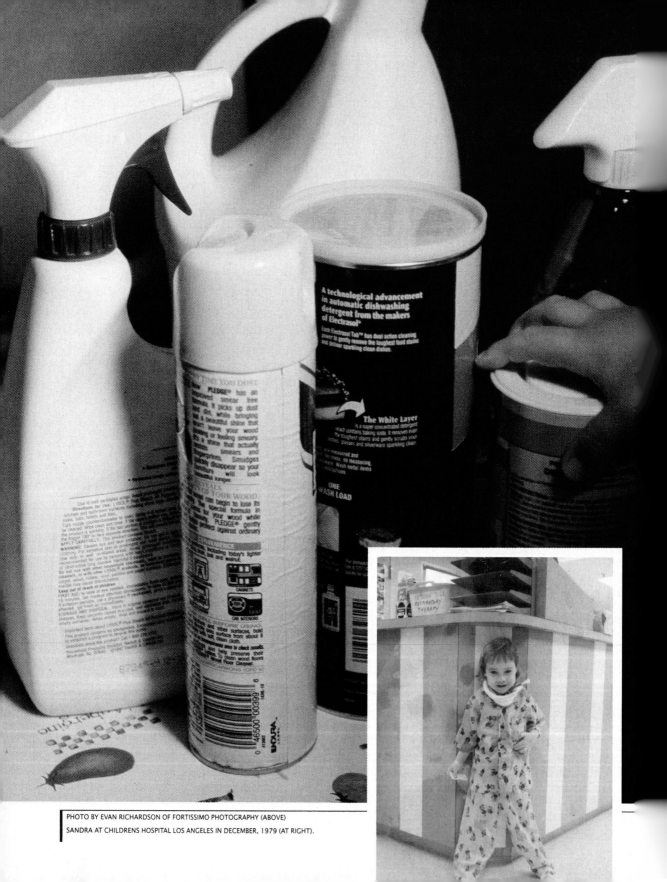

PHOTO BY EVAN RICHARDSON OF FORTISSIMO PHOTOGRAPHY (ABOVE)
SANDRA AT CHILDRENS HOSPITAL LOS ANGELES IN DECEMBER, 1979 (AT RIGHT).

Consequences Can Last a Lifetime

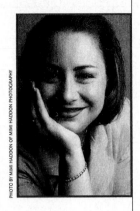

When I was 2½ years old, my dad went out for the evening and I was home with a sitter. Somehow I managed to get an outdoor storage cabinet open and drank DRANO. The sitter had me drink milk and induced vomiting. When my dad arrived three hours later, I was sleeping and my dad noticed purple blisters on my lips. He rushed me to a local emergency room and the doctors advised us to return within thirty days for my first surgery. This was to stretch my esophagus to make some repairs. However, during the surgery the doctor punctured my esophagus into my lung, so I was rushed to Childrens Hospital Los Angeles.

The subsequent surgeries to correct my esophagus resulted in being hospitalized for three-month intervals on numerous occasions. During the extensive surgeries I used a gastrointestinal tube to eat and then later graduated to baby food for some time. Luckily, I am doing well and have surgeries every year to stretch the esophagus to pass food comfortably. I now have a son of my own and because of my experience I take every precaution possible and I am always aware of my son's surroundings.

—*Sandra Kerans-Arlotti*

A CLOSER LOOK

Dr. Kenneth Geller, *Head, Division of Otolaryngology, Childrens Hospital Los Angeles, and Associate Professor of Otolaryngology, Keck School of Medicine, University of Southern California*
With the development of "child-proof" caps on caustic liquids and solids, the number of devastating ingestions has declined. Unfortunately, these still occur because of careless handling, especially around children. Children are often attracted to hazardous substances because they look like candy or soda. Therefore, extra precautions must be taken, including always closing a bottle even if it will be re-opened shortly; storing containers in a locked cabinet, and keeping products in their original container. Following these simple tips can prevent years of suffering.

Household chemicals are commonly used by adults, but pose the greatest poisoning threat to children. All household chemicals should be stored in a locked container that children cannot reach. Don't be fooled by environmentally friendly products; even though the products may prove less toxic, a great deal of permanent damage can still be done. Finally, try to only purchase products that have a childproof cap; although not completely child resistant, this safety feature does put time on your side.

Symptoms of Poisoning

Ingested	*Inhaled*	*Absorbed*
• Nausea and/or vomiting	• Headache	• Irregular breathing
• Change in breathing	• Difficulty breathing	• Abnormal pulse
• Diarrhea	• Dizziness	• Headache
• Unconsciousness	• Unconsciousness	• Skin or eye irritations

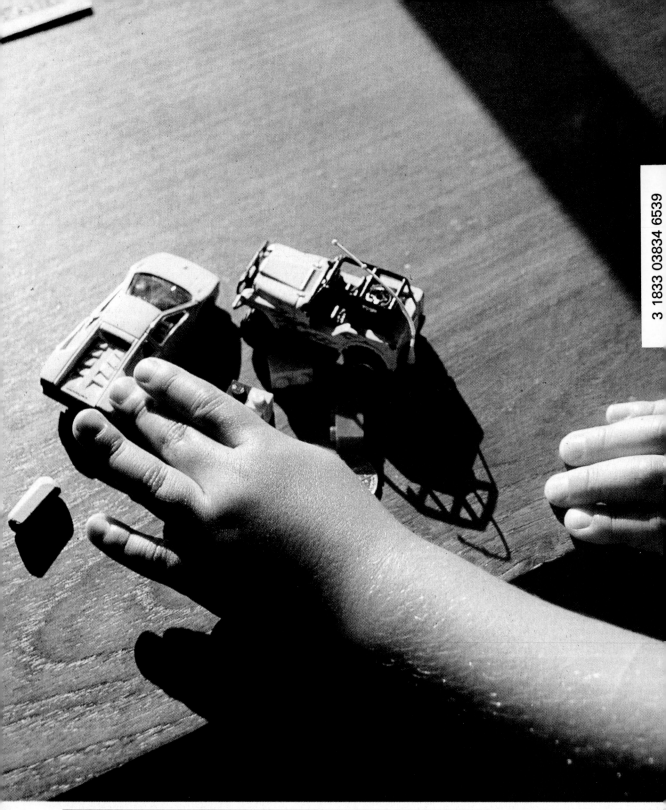

PHOTO BY EVAN RICHARDSON OF FORTISSIMO PHOTOGRAPHY

An Object Lesson

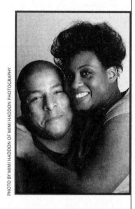

One of the scariest sounds in the world, especially to a parent, is the sound of a child choking. Knowing what to do can make the difference between your child living and dying. Our son, Eric, was two and getting into everything, when one day he began choking. He had found a rusty screw on the ground and put it in his mouth. We immediately called 911. We tried but were unable to dislodge the screw from his throat ourselves. Within a few short minutes, Eric's lips started turning blue. Fortunately, the paramedics were able to successfully perform CPR.

Eric is fine today, but the lessons we learned will last a lifetime. We are even more careful now to check for small items that might be lying around. Childproofing your house is an ongoing effort. You always say "this won't happen to me," but it can. All parents and guardians need to be prepared for the possibility of your child choking on something and know how to help when it happens.

—Katina and Emery Washington

A CLOSER LOOK

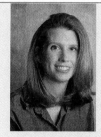

Dr. Karen McVeigh, *Attending Physician, Pediatric Intensive Care Unit, Childrens Hospital Los Angeles, and Assistant Professor of Pediatrics, Keck School of Medicine, University of Southern California*
Keep small objects away from infants and young children, who are at special risk for choking—the most common cause of accidental death under the age of one year. Inhaling an object can block the airways. Coughing, difficulty breathing, inability to talk and a change in skin color can all indicate partial blockage. With complete blockage, the child loses consciousness within minutes.

Dr. Debra Don, *Attending Physician, Division of Otolaryngology, Childrens Hospital Los Angeles, and Assistant Professor, Pediatric Otolaryngology/Head and Neck Surgery, Keck School of Medicine, University of Southern California*
Food is responsible for most cases of choking in children. Avoid giving infants any food that requires chewing until they are at least eight months old and have teeth. And don't feed children under four years of age hard, smooth foods or round food, which can lodge in their windpipe. The "forbidden" list includes peanuts, popcorns, hot dogs, carrot and celery cut into circles or sticks, grapes, and hard candies.

Choking and Suffocation Hazards for Young Children

Toys	Foods	Small Objects
• Marbles	• Hot dogs	• Pins and safety pins
• Balloons	• Grapes	• Toothpicks
• Dress-up jewelry	• Gum	• Tacks
• Plastic bags	• Lollipops	• Jewelry
• Any toy less than 1½ inches in diameter	• Carrots, celery, and other raw vegetables	• Coins
• Game tokens and pieces	• Peanuts	• Crayons
• Jacks	• Popcorn	• Nails
• Toy chest with no air holes	• Olives	• Pencils and pens
	• Hard candy and lemon drops	• Staples

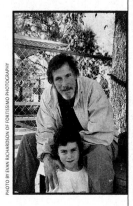

Bathroom Safety

The bathroom in your home can be a very dangerous place for adults and children. My family and I learned this firsthand. My son Julius was just becoming potty trained and still had to be reminded to go to the bathroom. Early one morning, I had just taken a shower and the floor was a little wet. We had what I thought were sufficient area rugs in place. When Julius came running into the bathroom, he didn't have a chance. He hit the wet floor and his feet went to the left, while his head continued to the right. His face hit the edge of the toilet bowl, opening a gash near his left eyebrow. The cut required six stitches. Although the injury wasn't terribly serious, I'll never forget having to hold my son down while the doctor cleaned and stitched the cut.

I've learned a great lesson in all this. Now I make a conscious effort to slow down and take care to dry the bathroom floor after showering. Plus, we've put down an adequate number of rugs to decrease the likelihood of a similar injury ever occurring again.

—*Mark Metcalf*

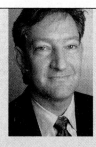

A CLOSER LOOK

Dr. Alan Nager, *Director, Emergency and Transport Medicine, Childrens Hospital Los Angeles, and Assistant Professor of Pediatrics, Keck School of Medicine, University of Southern California*
Trauma is the most under-recognized public health problem in the nation today. Bathrooms, although not high on the list of hazardous environments at first glance, have inherent dangers. As a favorite climbing and play area for young children, a variety of injuries can occur, including head injuries, broken bones, near drownings, ingestions, and hot water burns. The following safety guidelines will help eliminate unnecessary injuries:

- Always supervise children in the bathroom.
- Never walk away for such things as answering the door or telephone or getting a towel, even for a few seconds.
- Wipe up spills immediately.
- Bathe young children using appropriate bath seats.
- With older children, keep the door unlocked at all times in order to gain entry should an injury occur.
- Keep toilet seats down at all times and utilize toilet seat safety clips if young children are in the home.
- Always test water temperature before bathing your child. The temperature should be between 90 to 120 degrees Fahrenheit.

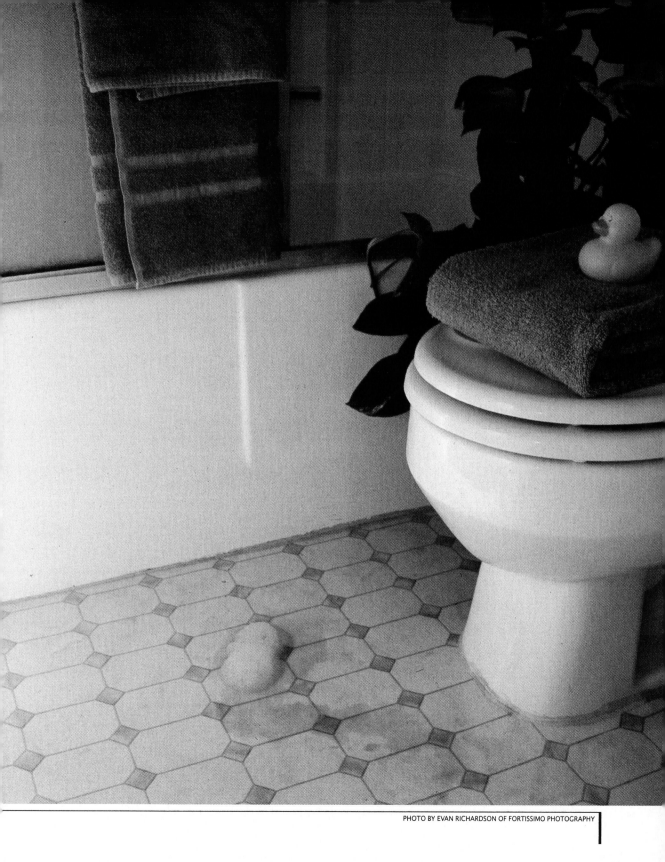

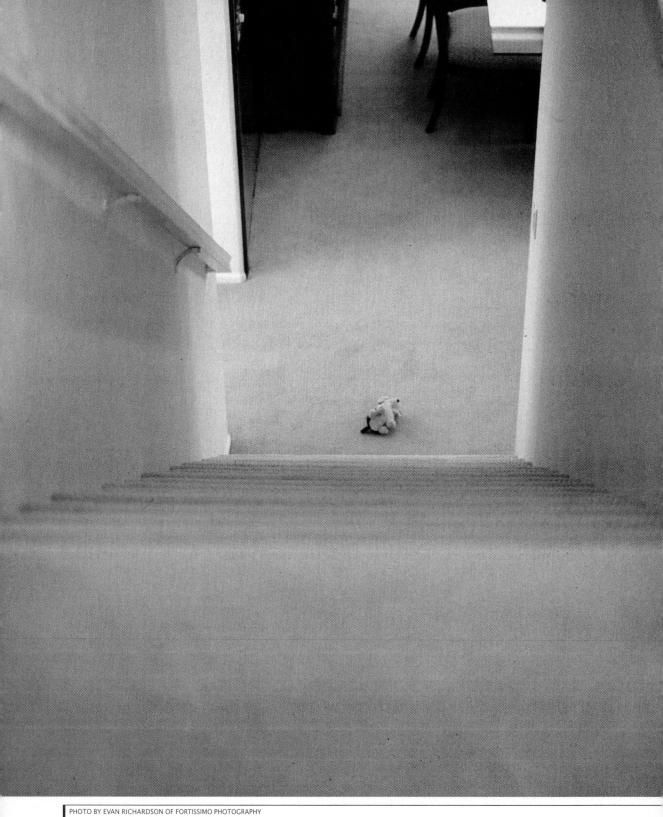

Keep the Gate Closed

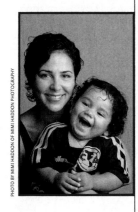

Most people realize that stairs can be dangerous terrain for toddlers. That's why our family installed a safety gate at the top of the stairs in our home. But taking such a precaution isn't always enough—something I learned the hard way.

My ten-month-old, Christian, was upstairs in his walker one morning—it was just a typical day. I turned my back for just a moment and heard him fall. He tumbled down seventeen steps. The safety gate had been left open. I immediately called my mother who drove us to the emergency room. We were lucky. By some miracle, Christian suffered only bumps and bruises. As his mother, however, I continue to question why I did not notice that the gate at the top of the stairs was not closed. The outcome could have been so much worse. Anything can happen in an instant—even when you've done what you thought was the "right thing" to prevent it.

—Peggy Rodriguez

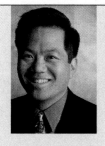

A CLOSER LOOK

Dr. Calvin Lowe, *Medical Director, Childrens Emergency Transport, Attending Physician, Department of Emergency and Transport Medicine, Childrens Hospital Los Angeles, and Assistant Professor of Pediatrics, Keck School of Medicine, University of Southern California*

Without proper safety equipment, infants and toddlers can easily fall down a flight of stairs. Install gates at the top and bottom of a stairway. At the top, never use a pressure gate because children can topple them; instead, attach the gate to the wall. Keep stairs clear of objects, as young children love to run up and down stairs with reckless energy. In addition, do not allow infants and young children to use a walker.

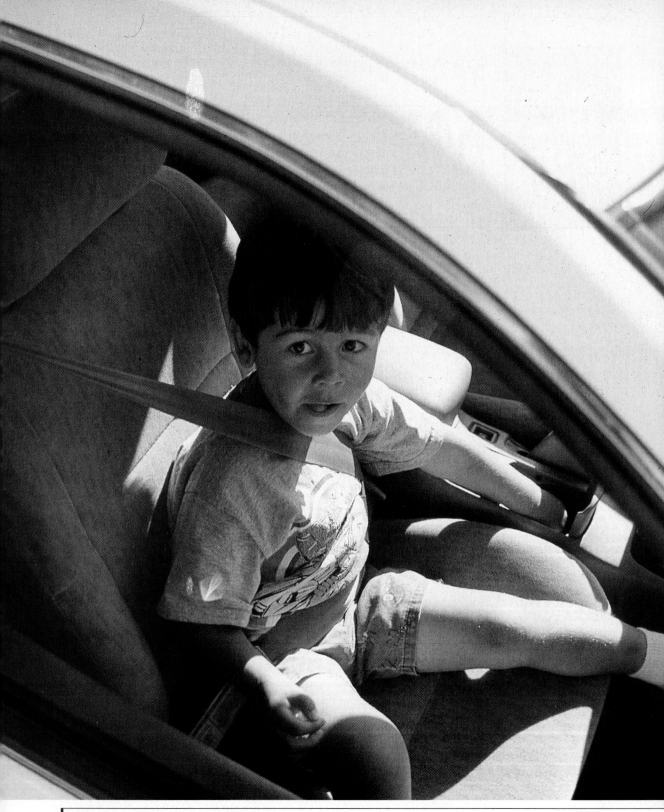

vehicles

E very state requires that infants be placed in child safety seats and children ride buckled up. However, more children are killed and injured in car crashes than from any other type of injury [6]. Every child riding in a vehicle should be placed in a car seat, unless the child is big enough for a shoulder belt to lie across the shoulder rather than the neck or throat, the lap belt to lie flat across the hips, and the child's knees bend easily over the edge of the seat [6]. There are four main types of car seats: infant-only, convertible seats, forward-facing seats, and boosters. No one car seat is the best. The most appropriate car seat is the one that fits your child's size and weight, and can be installed correctly in your car [6].

In addition to motor vehicle safety, parents need to be especially cautious when using bicycles, motorcycles, and all-terrain vehicles (ATVs). Many children are seriously injured using these wheeled vehicles.

Each story in this section focuses on safety associated with wheeled vehicles. The stories are true and each provides specific safety advice for a different type of vehicle.

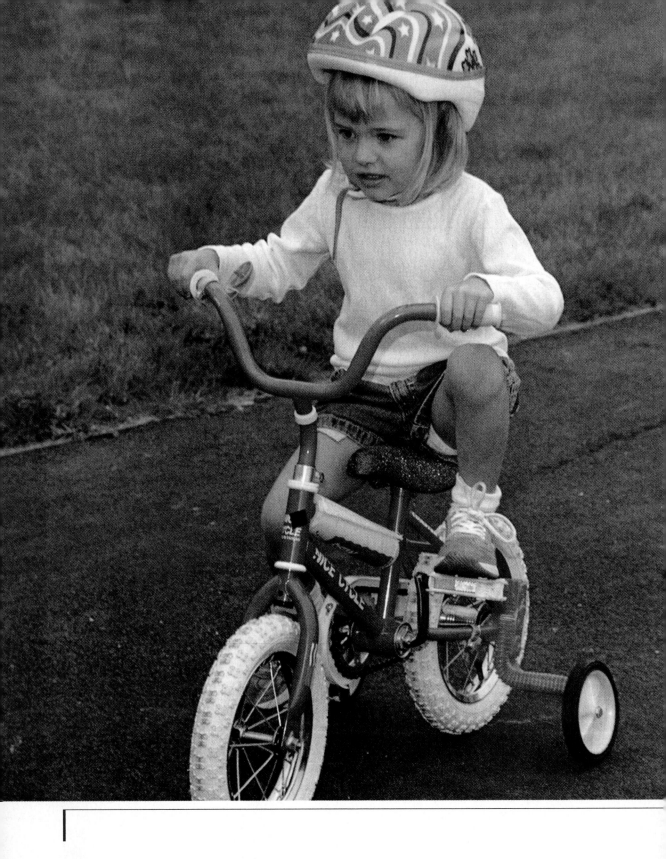

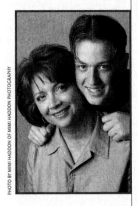

A Lifesaving Helmet

Our eleven-year-old son Peter's favorite thing to do was to ride his bike. He had been riding for some time, and we were both gaining confidence in his growing skills. The street was busy that day but not unusually so; he had ridden it many times before. Suddenly—in a blink of the eye—Peter was struck by a car. His injuries were so serious he had to be airlifted by helicopter to Childrens Hospital Los Angeles, where physicians, nurses, and other personnel in the emergency room immediately went to work. In the hospital, he began the slow process of healing. You never believe something like this is going to happen to you. But when it does, be glad that those services are there for you. The one saving grace of that day—our son was wearing a helmet. I'm confident that bicycle helmet saved Peter's life.

I advise any parent to always enforce the use of safety equipment—no matter what your child's age. Whether your child is riding a bicycle, tricycle, or ride-on vehicle, he or she should wear a helmet at all times. Without that one piece of equipment, our son might not be here today.

—Denice and Bill Beal

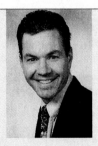

A CLOSER LOOK

Dr. J. Duncan Phillips, *Associate Professor of Surgery, Section of Pediatric Surgery, School of Medicine, University of North Carolina at Chapel Hill, and Attending Surgeon, University of North Carolina Hospitals (formerly at Childrens Hospital Los Angeles)*

Peter sustained multiple life-threatening injuries, including a collapsed right lung, a broken leg with protruding bone, and bleeding in his abdominal cavity. It is nearly certain that he avoided a serious or even fatal brain injury because he was wearing a helmet. The Centers for Disease Control and Prevention (CDC) have estimated that as many as 184 deaths and 116,000 head injuries might be prevented annually if all bicycle riders wore helmets [7].

Here are some simple safety tips for children and adults:

- Wear a protective helmet and age-appropriate safety protection.
- Ride in well-lit, designated bicycle paths or lanes.
- Wear reflective clothing at night and have a secure light and bicycle reflectors.
- Take a bicycle safety class.

Safety helmets should also be worn when riding tricycles, Big Wheels, go-carts, and battery-operated vehicles.

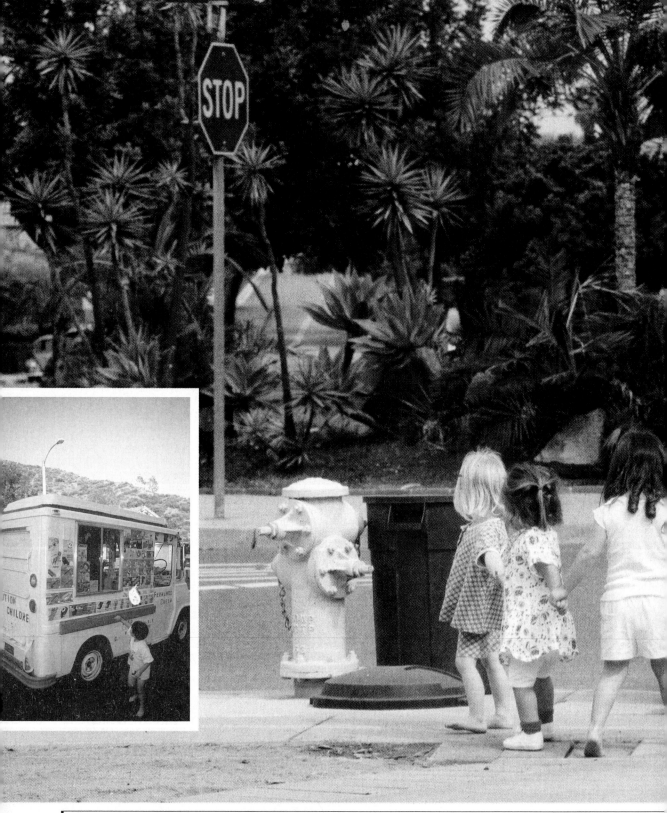

Danger at the Sidewalk

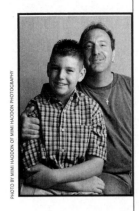

Adam had just finished in-line skating at the local skate park with four of his best friends. Everyone decided to cross the street and get some food at Burger King. The boys were standing at the street corner waiting for the light to change when a young driver approached and lost control of the vehicle he was driving. The car struck a light pole and then ricocheted into the boys. Adam, who was eleven at the time, was struck and thrown thirty feet. All of his friends were also struck.

I am an Emergency Medical Technician (EMT) and arrived on the scene within five minutes of the accident. I can't begin to describe how it felt to see my child on the ground bleeding and asking me if he was going to die. Adam was flown to Holy Cross Medical Center and then taken by ambulance to Childrens Hospital Los Angeles because of concerns over respiratory difficulties. He was in the hospital for five days, suffered three broken ribs, and had glass in his face and arms. Luckily, he was wearing his helmet. His helmet decreased the severity of his injuries evidenced by the dents and scratches to his helmet and not to his head. However, as a family we are still paying because the insurance limits carried by the driver were so low. In addition, all of Adam's friends were severely injured.

As parents, we would both like to ask all other parents to encourage their young drivers to drive carefully because too many lose their lives or radically change the lives of others.

—*Mark and Lynda Woolley*

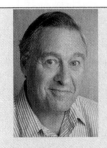

A CLOSER LOOK

David Niven, Jr., *Chairman of See a Child, Save a Child*
A pedestrian is killed in a vehicle crash on average every 101 minutes and one is injured every 8 minutes. Twenty-five percent of pedestrians killed are between the ages of five and nine; 30 percent of pedalcyclists killed are between five and fifteen. Forty-four percent of all pedestrian fatalities under the age of 16 occur between 4 P.M. and 8 P.M.; 65 percent of all pedestrian deaths occur when it's dark, while 78 percent occur at non-intersections [8]. I had the horrifying experience of witnessing a child killed by a car at around 5 P.M. last year. I am extremely proud to have created the See A Child, Save A Child pedestrian and pedalcyclist safety kit. Each kit contains twenty adhesive reflective stickers that will help make your children and those in your neighborhood more visible.

Dr. Hossein Mahour, *Director, Trauma Program, Childrens Hospital Los Angeles, and Professor of Surgery, Keck School of Medicine, University of Southern California*
Another often overlooked killer of children is the ice cream truck. Many children are seriously injured or killed each year. Parents should always supervise children when approaching an ice cream truck, and never allow children to run after or toward a vehicle.

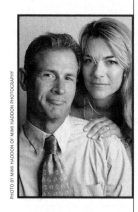

Trust Your Instincts

It was late at night when we received the telephone call all parents dread—our son had been injured in a motor vehicle accident. Henry, fifteen, had gone on a fishing trip with his friends. There were four boys in one pickup truck. Because all four could not ride in the truck cab, the boys drew sticks to see who would ride in the back. Henry lost and reluctantly agreed to ride in the truck bed, even though his instincts told him it wasn't the safest thing to do. He was riding in the back when the driver lost control and his truck rolled over. With the force of the rollover, Henry was ejected fifty feet, landing away from the road. The emergency response unit had a difficult time finding him, losing precious moments. Henry was airlifted to the hospital, where after extensive examinations to his spinal column, he was immobilized preventing probable paralysis. He is now doing well and has even entered college early—but that phone call still haunts us.

As a parent, you can never talk too much about safety. Teach your children to trust their instincts and avoid any situation they feel is dangerous.

—*Carol and John Blunt*

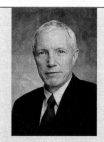

A CLOSER LOOK

Dr. Gordon McComb, *Head, Division of Neurosurgery, Childrens Hospital Los Angeles, and Professor of Neurological Surgery, Keck School of Medicine, University of Southern California*
Because most childhood injuries result from motor vehicle accidents, prevention is the key. A broken limb can heal, but a brain or spinal cord injury can produce a lifelong neurological deficit. Protecting our children requires the use of a properly installed car seat, wearing a seatbelt, and safe vehicle habits. Never take chances.

Efrain Garza Fuentes, *Ed.D., Director, Patient and Family Services, Childrens Hospital Los Angeles, and Voluntary Faculty Member, Keck School of Medicine, University of Southern California*
Ability to comprehend verbal communications and commands will vary greatly depending on your child's age. But there is a constant that runs through the entire childhood spectrum called self-esteem. Children who feel strong can face the challenges, confront the obstacles, and effectively problem solve the thorny situations they will likely face. Self-esteem will give them the tools to make the right choice when faced with an unsafe situation, even if means calling mom or dad in the middle of the night.

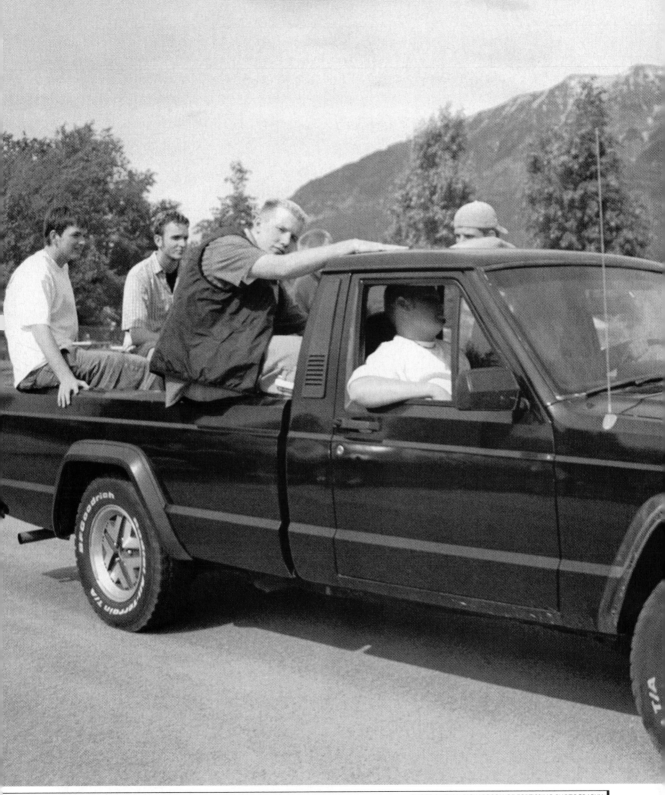

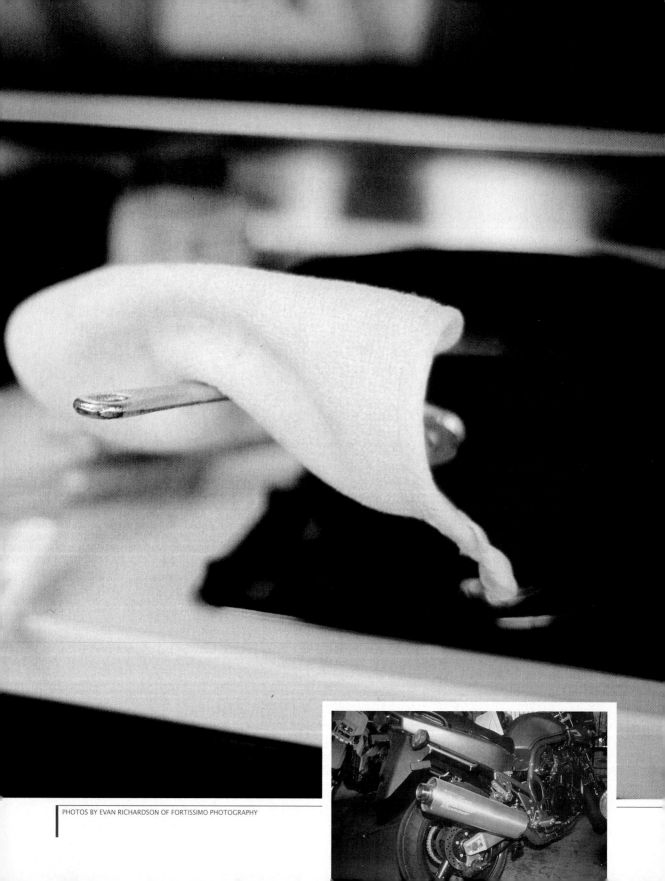

Don't Get Burned

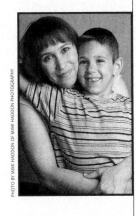

Our son, Sam, who was seven, often went dirt bike riding with his dad, and we had been careful to purchase all the special gear including boots. One time, after riding all day, his group was taking a break when the kids decided to ride around the camp. Because the riding was only going to be around the camp and all the adults were present, Sam did not put on his gear. Rather he started riding wearing only his shorts and a top. After about five minutes, Sam's bike lost its traction and fell over on Sam. Sam was trapped under his dirt bike and all the time the bike was on him the exhaust pipe was burning his leg. His uncle threw the bike off of him but not before his leg was severely burned. Once Sam returned from the trip, I immediately contacted our pediatrician who referred us to the hospital. Although Sam's leg was severely burned no surgery was necessary. We have been to the doctor four times since the injury took place, and have spent huge sums of money on gauze, which is not covered by medical insurance.

Safety equipment is only useful if you use it. As a parent, it is your responsibility to ensure that your child uses the safety equipment every time—no excuses.

—*Donna Stringer*

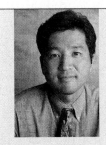

A CLOSER LOOK

Dr. Tao Ho Kim, *Attending Physician, Division of Plastic Surgery, Childrens Hospital Los Angeles, and Assistant Professor of Plastic Surgery, Keck School of Medicine, University of Southern California*
Burn injuries are very common among infants and children, and happen quickly. All burn injuries are preventable. The most common sources of burn injuries are boiling water, hot soup, hot tap water, and hot machines or appliances. Appropriate precautions should always be taken such as maintaining a proper water heater temperature of 120 degrees Fahrenheit and keeping pot handles and hot devices from being grabbed. Burn injuries are extremely painful and can lead to temporary or permanent disfigurement and deformity.

Children receive burns from a variety of sources:

- Stoves: Always use the back burners.
- Hot drinks: Don't leave them unattended and push the container to the center of a table.
- Electrical cords: Check for worn cords.
- Bath water: Always test the temperature of the bathwater before placing a child in the bathtub.

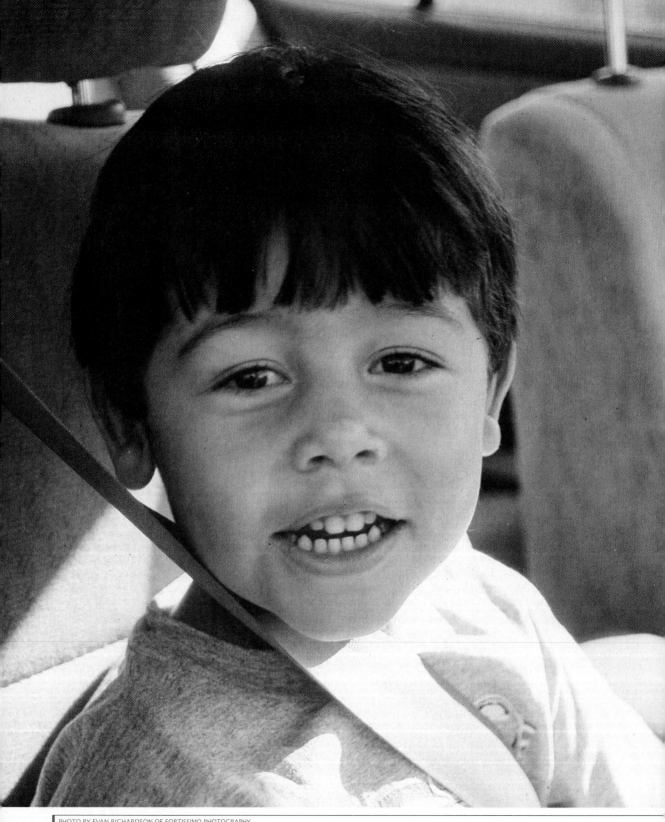

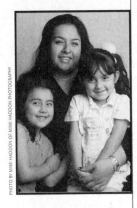

Car Seats: Safety for Kids Up to the Age of Eight

Our entire family was in the car enjoying an outing when another driver ran a red light and struck our car. Our car spun around and hit a water pump at a gas station. As our car was struck, Elizabeth, who is three, was thrown forward and hit the back of the seat in front of her. As a result she lost two teeth and cut her gums and lips. Elizabeth was not in a car seat, but was wearing a seat belt. Therefore, she was not restrained and her injuries could have been much worse than they were. In contrast, Matthew, who is one, was in a car seat and sustained no injuries at all. An ambulance responded to the accident and Elizabeth was taken to the hospital. At the hospital, an x-ray of Elizabeth's jaw and skull revealed that there was no brain injury or concussion. We were very lucky. In order to repair the damage to Elizabeth's teeth, gums, and lips we had to seek a pediatric dentist. We are still working with the dentist and are hopeful. Unfortunately, the emotional wounds take much longer to heal. Elizabeth feels angry at the other driver and feels scared whenever she is in the car, constantly asking, "Are we going to crash again?" Although not every motor vehicle accident can be avoided, using the right safety equipment can reduce serious injuries.

—*Christina and Ancelmo Perez*

A CLOSER LOOK

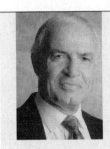

Dr. G. Hossein Mahour, *Director, Trauma Program, Childrens Hospital Los Angeles, and Professor of Surgery, Keck School of Medicine, University of Southern California*
Of all the pediatric trauma patients treated at Childrens Hospital Los Angeles, 65 percent have received their injuries from some incident with a vehicle—as a passenger, pedestrian, bicyclist, or as a young driver. Injury prevention can be divided into three steps:

1. Primary prevention is the prevention of the incident from occurring such as stopping on a yellow light and not running a red light.
2. Secondary prevention is the mitigation of severe injuries with the use of safety equipment such as car seats and seat belts.
3. Tertiary prevention is the reduction of the long-term effects of an injury through the availability of a level one trauma center such as Childrens Hospital Los Angeles.

Dr. Jose Polido, *Assistant Clinic Director, Residency Director Pediatric Dentistry, Childrens Hospital Los Angeles, and Assistant Professor of Clinical Dentistry, University of Southern California, School of Dentistry*
Being prepared for dental trauma is part of effective prevention. The use of mouth guards can prevent damage to the teeth. Know that if a permanent tooth is completely knocked out of its socket it should be replanted immediately by a dentist or kept in cold milk until replantation. With baby teeth, preventing disturbances to the underlying developing permanent teeth is the key. In both situations, timely treatment is essential.

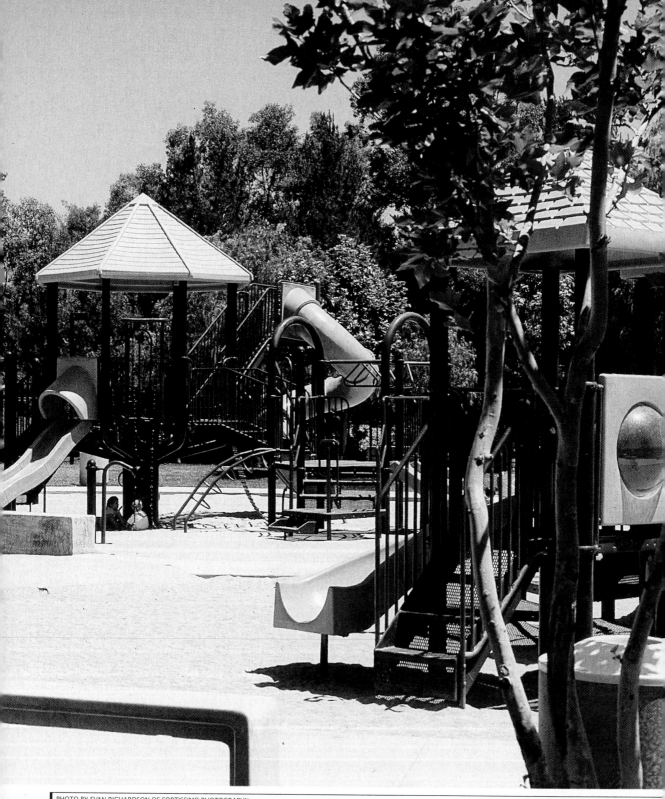

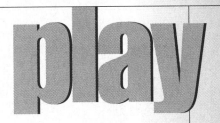

E ach year, approximately 211,000 preschool and elementary children receive emergency room care for injuries that occurred on playground equipment [9]. The majority of injuries result from swings, slides, and climbing equipment. Play is the work of children and, therefore, every effort must be made to ensure the safety of our children at play. As a parent, that includes inspection of playground equipment at home, school, and public recreation areas you frequently use. It also requires that parents be willing to object to dangerous equipment, discontinue use of the equipment, and notify the appropriate authorities.

Parents must also take an active role in safety when a child is involved in organized sports activities. Find out what safety equipment is recommended for the sports your child plays and insist that the equipment be used every time—no excuses.

Toy selection is also critical. Look for age-appropriate toys. Toys for children three and younger should not have small parts and should be too large to swallow. Toys also should not come apart easily or have removable button eyes or beanbag fillings.

Finally, be a good role model. Always wear your own safety equipment and your child is likely to follow your example.

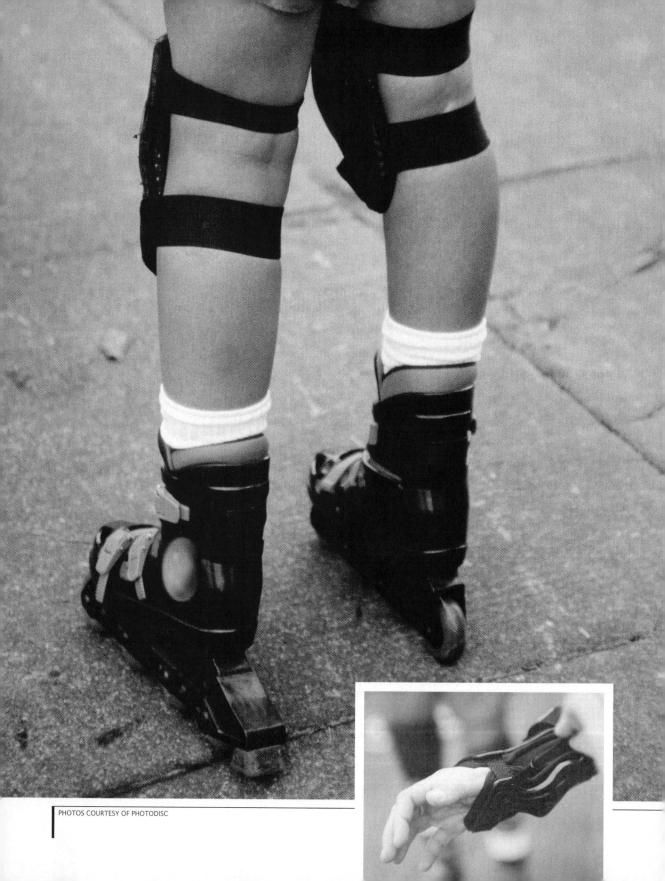

Safety Equipment First

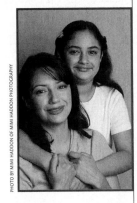

Because I work in a hospital, I know the importance of safety equipment in preventing injuries. However, it's often hard to enforce the rules about wearing safety equipment with your own kids. They complain the equipment is too heavy, it takes too long to put on, they'll only be out for a short time, or they don't look "cool" enough wearing it. Ignore their complaints.

One afternoon, my nine-year-old daughter, Sharen, went in-line skating with her father without wearing any elbow or wrist guards. A pebble got stuck in one of her wheels while accelerating and she was instantly propelled forward. When she landed, she broke both her arms. Imagine your child with his or her arms in a cast—how hard is it to bathe, go to school, dress, even eat. The early days after the injury were uncomfortable and often painful for Sharen.

I am happy to report Sharen has recovered fully. Equally important, our family has learned an important lesson: Safety gear can't do anything to protect you unless you use it. We all now use the appropriate safety equipment every time, no matter what sport we're playing or for how long. I encourage every family to do the same.

—Maria Angulo

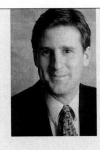

A CLOSER LOOK

Dr. Robert Kay, *Attending Physician, Division of Orthopedic Surgery, Childrens Hospital Los Angeles, and Assistant Professor of Orthopedic Surgery, Keck School of Medicine, University of Southern California*

In-line skating is a good source of fun and exercise. But follow certain rules to stay safe.

- Always wear safety gear: helmet, elbow pads, wrist guards, and knee pads.
- Wear reflective clothing after dark or near dusk.
- Do not wear a Walkman.
- Do not in-line skate in the street.
- When learning, don't skate downhill as you might have difficulty stopping.
- Always be careful around driveways.

Causes of similar injuries

- Rollerskating
- Skateboarding
- Bicycle riding

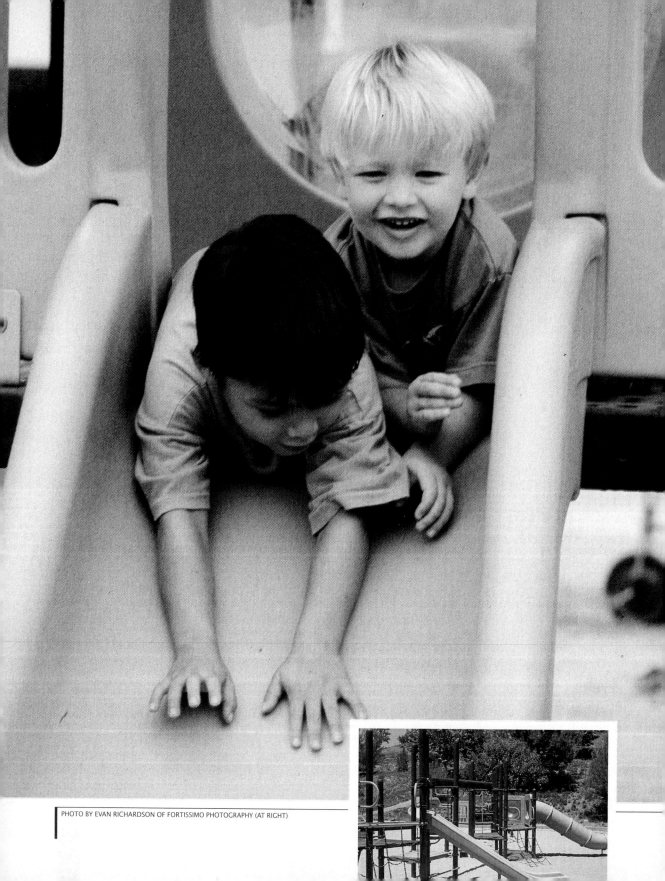

Playground Safety

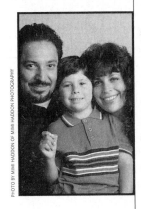

We hadn't been away from our three-year old son, Cristian, a day since he was born. We were nervous, but confident about the child care we had arranged. The events that occurred while we were out of town irrevocably altered our lives. On the day of our departure, Cristian was taken to the park by the babysitter, just as we ourselves had often done. He enjoyed sliding and was now able to climb the ladder up to the slide by himself and slide down. This time, things took a tragic turn. Cristian was at the top of a six-foot slide when he lost his footing and toppled to the hard packed dirt below. His skull was fractured and he was in a coma for two weeks. Once he recovered from the coma, he was left with a brain injury that will affect him the rest of his life. He continues to receive rehabilitation. We feel blessed he has recovered so well, however; the financial and emotional consequences never seem to end.

We urge all parents to carefully watch their children on playgrounds. Although we as parents try hard to be careful at playgrounds and parks the unexpected can happen, be aware of such hidden dangers as inadequate ground cover. Even if it means upsetting your child, leaving a playground is better than risking injury.

—*Kristine and Gerardo Alvarez*

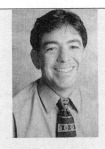

A CLOSER LOOK

Dr. Luis Montes, *Medical Director of the Rehabilitation Department, and Assistant Professor of Pediatrics, Keck School of Medicine, University of Southern California*

Nothing is more important than the choice of ground cover to reduce the severity of injuries from falls. Natural grass or asphalt surfaces are inappropriate for playgrounds and do not sufficiently absorb the impact of a fall. Wood mulch, sand or synthetic surfaces are acceptable as long as they are sufficiently thick to absorb the energy from a fall. The higher the potential fall the thicker the ground cover should be. A ten- to twelve-inch thick layer of loose-fill material is recommended when the height of the fall would be no greater than six feet for a school-age child and five feet or less for younger children.

Guidelines for the design and layout of playground equipment are available in *The Handbook for Public Playground Safety, 1991,* and can be obtained by contacting the U.S. Consumer Product Safety Commission.

Keeping Safe on the Playground

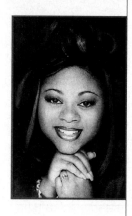

I remember when I was about seven or eight getting hurt by the swings at the playground. It all happened because I really was not paying attention to my surroundings.

I had just gotten off the merry-go-round and was a bit dizzy from the ride and was headed towards an empty swing to continue my fun. As I walked dizzily to the swings, all I can really remember is a scream warning me to "Watch out!" One of my little girlfriends had seen what was just about to happen and she tried in vain to warn me.

There was this big kid from junior high school who was swinging very high. He was even standing up! He probably didn't see me, but he should have been swinging more carefully. But, I must bear part of the blame because I should have been looking where I was walking.

When the swing hit me, it knocked the breath completely from me! Everybody was screaming! Blood was streaming from my mouth. When I awoke, an ambulance attendant could see that I was responding and no bones were broken. A later checkup by the doctor gave me good news. I was going to be OK. Now the lesson to be learned is—always be aware of your surroundings on the playground.

—*Countess Vaughn*

A CLOSER LOOK

All children should know the rules for the safe use of playground equipment. Take a few minutes to review the following rules with your child in case they have not received proper instruction at daycare or school:

- Wait until the swing comes to a complete stop before getting on or off
- Only one child should be on each swing at any time.
- Always sit on the swing seat—no standing
- Hold on with both hands
- Steer clear of moving swings
- Do not use swings that look broken or worn

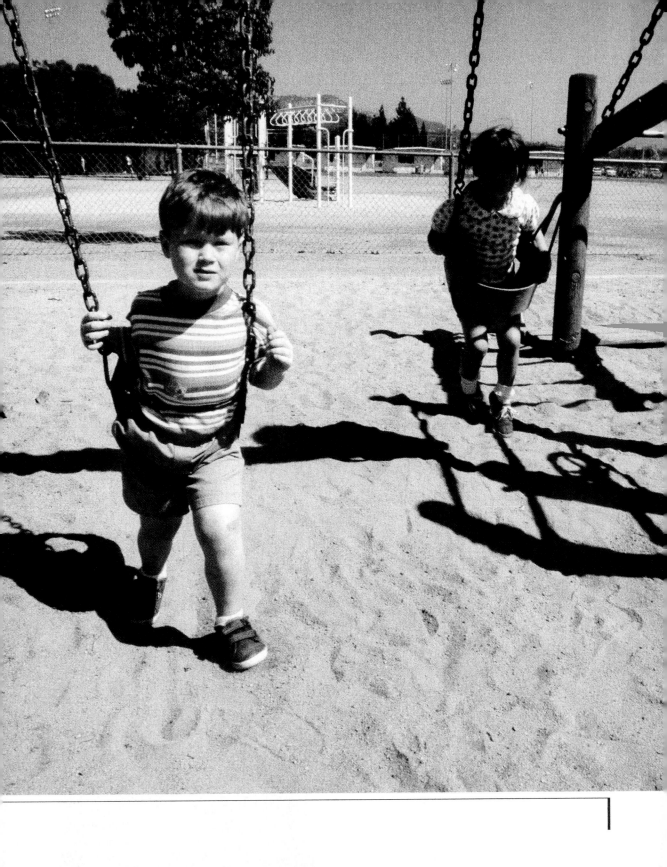

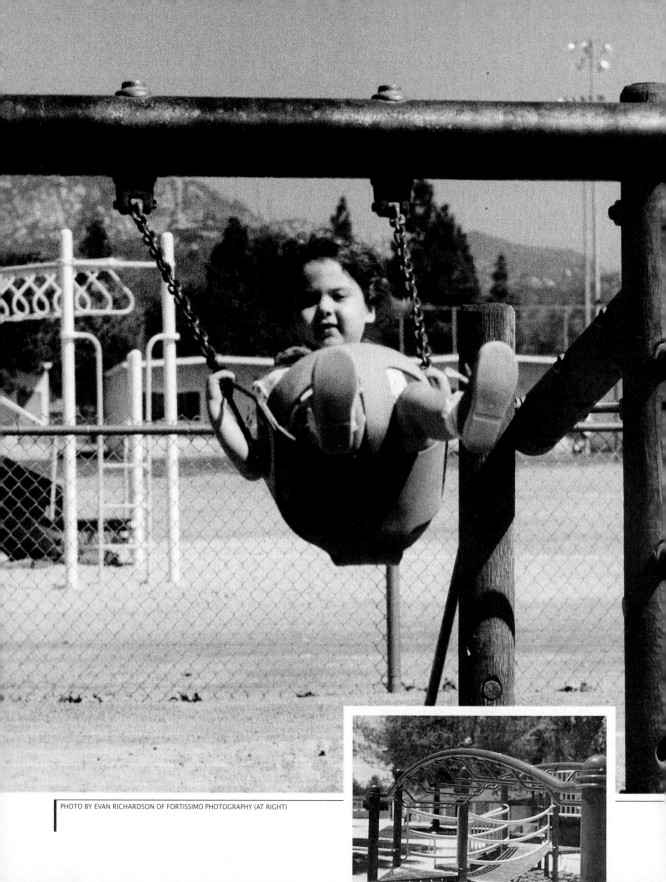

PHOTO BY EVAN RICHARDSON OF FORTISSIMO PHOTOGRAPHY (AT RIGHT)

Consequences of Risky Play

As a parent, the most frightening call you can receive is one informing you that your child has been injured. We sent our five-year old son Attila to school on what seemed like an average day. We never expected to get the phone call we received. Attila and his friends always enjoy playing outside at recess. On this particular day, they decided to play on the monkey bars, competing with one another to see who could cross them without falling. They were clapping for each other as each of them made it across. As Attila was crossing, one of the boys jokingly pulled his fingers off the bars. Unable to reach the next bar, Attila fell to the ground, landing on his elbow. He was joking with his friends at first when he fell, but then he realized he was in pain. When we got the phone call telling us he had been hurt, we rushed to the school. We took him to Children's Hospital in Washington D.C. to have his arm examined and x-rayed. Unfortunately, our son had broken his elbow and needed surgery to repair the damage. Attila had been hurt before at the playground, falling off the slide, but he had never broken any bones.

The playground at his school was new and the ground underneath the equipment is fairly soft, so we never thought he would be hurt so badly. We know when children play with each other, accidents will happen, but we hope that was the last of the injuries on the playground that Attila will have to face.

—*Margit and Istvan Toth*

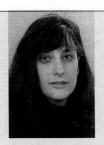

A CLOSER LOOK

Dr. Terry Adirim, *Attending, Emergency Department, Children's National Medical Center, Washington, D.C.*

Falls are the most common mechanism, or cause, of injury in children. Most falls lead to minor injuries, but falls from heights increase the risk for more serious injuries. The most common injury resulting from a fall is a fracture. The key to reducing the chance of fractures is ensuring that the surface surrounding playground equipment is designed to absorb the impact of a fall.

Avoid asphalt, concrete, grass and soil surfaces under playground equipment and choose a loose fill, such as hardwood fiber mulch or chips, pea gravel, fine sand, or shredded rubber. Loose fill should be maintained at a depth of 12 inches and extend a minimum of 6 feet in all directions around stationary equipment. [From Falls Fact Sheet, the National SAFEKIDS Campaign, www.safekids.org/fact99/falls99]

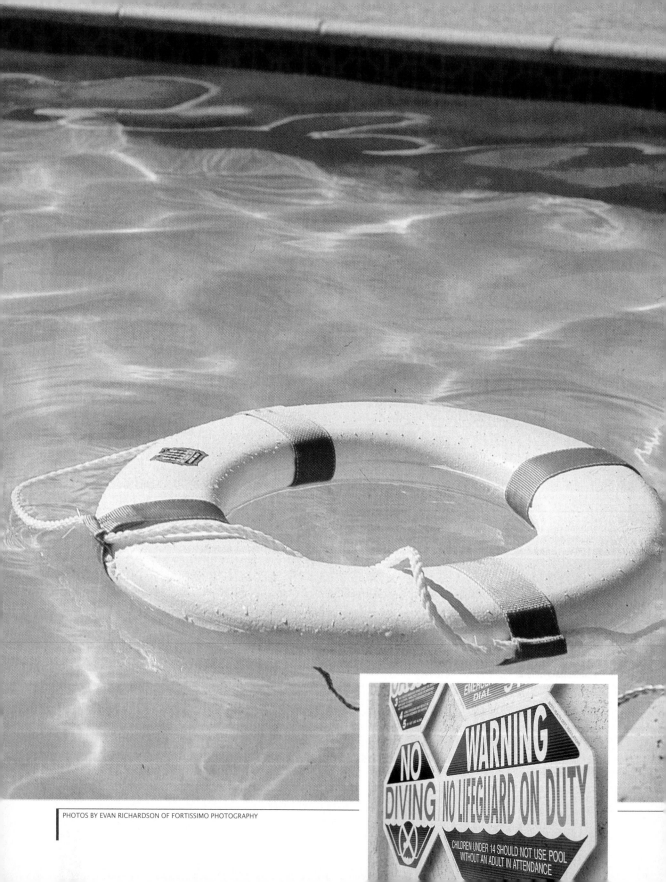

EMERGENCY
DIAL

NO DIVING

WARNING
NO LIFEGUARD ON DUTY

CHILDREN UNDER 14 SHOULD NOT USE POOL
WITHOUT AN ADULT IN ATTENDANCE

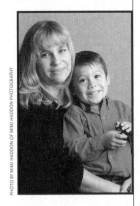

A Near Drowning

As a social worker, I pride myself on teaching other parents how to take care of their children on a daily basis. That professional knowledge did not give me immunity against the near drowning of my two-year-old son, Jovan. Our family has a backyard swimming pool. We understand the importance of pool safety and took the precaution of installing a pool net. On the day in question, Jovan was outside playing and I was watching him through the windows. The pool net was not on the pool and I went to the garage to get something from my car. When I returned I could not see Jovan. I rushed outside and found Jovan at the bottom of the pool—a horrifying image that haunts me to this day. As I pulled him out his body was limp and I laid him down on the concrete. I immediately called 911 and started CPR [cardiopulmonary resuscitation]. I don't know how I knew what to do, I had taken CPR twelve years ago but after performing CPR about ten times, Jovan started breathing on his own. The ambulance responded within three minutes and he was rushed to Childrens Hospital Los Angeles. He spent two nights in the hospital and returned home. Although he seems physically fine, he is still haunted by the event and has experienced nightmares.

I urge all parents to install safety equipment and use it every time. Most importantly, don't assume that if you step away for "just a minute" that nothing will happen. It only takes a second to change your life forever.

—*Marilyn Pulgar*

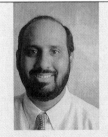

A CLOSER LOOK

Dr. Sajjad Yacoob, *Director, Undergraduate Medical Education, Childrens Hospital Los Angeles, Attending Physician, Division of General Pediatrics, Childrens Hospital Los Angeles, and Assistant Professor of Pediatrics, Keck School of Medicine, University of Southern California*

Drowning claims nearly 4,000 lives annually and it is the leading cause of accidental death in children one to four years old [10]. Children under five and adolescent boys are the highest risk groups for drowning and near drowning. Infants often drown in bathtubs or buckets, while home pools are the chief danger for children ages one to four. Older children and teens are at risk in lakes, ponds, rivers, or pools. Irreversible brain damage from a near drowning can occur when the brain is deprived of oxygen for as little as four minutes. Here are a few simple tips to prevent drowning and near drowning:

- Make sure there is constant adult supervision of young children playing in or near water or in bath tubs.
- A five-foot high, four-sided pool fence with a self-closing, self-latching gate should surround all pools.
- Children should wear approved personal flotation devices when on boats or in water.
- Learn CPR and update your training regularly.
- Use toilet lid locks when toddlers are in the house.
- Don't use five-gallon buckets or larger.
- **Always check the pool first if your child is missing; remember, seconds count!**

See the Appendix for additional water safety guidelines.

Root for School Safety

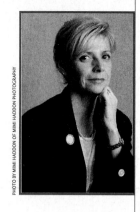

All kids love to attend athletic events and cheer for their teams. Even in this seemingly innocuous setting, parents need to be vigilant about safety. My fourteen-year-old daughter, Candice, was sitting in the bleachers observing a track and field practice at her high school—a place you'd assume is safe. Unfortunately, Candice was struck in the head with a discus. She was airlifted by helicopter to the hospital and subsequently underwent brain surgery. We were terrified because at first Candice did not recognize me or her dad and was disoriented and very combative. As her condition stabilized, she improved, but our family continues to suffer the aftereffects. I had to leave work without pay and still suffer from stress and lack of sleep. We are also in family/marriage counseling due to this traumatic event. Most of all, I question the circumstances and what I could have done to prevent the injury.

What I have learned is that you can't rely on a school or anyone else to secure your child's safety. You must be proactive and alert to unsafe situations and be willing to request that the school authorities improve them. Take time to visit your child's school. If you find any unsafe sports equipment or facilities, don't hesitate to speak up.

—*Katheryn Tizcareno*

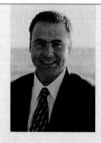

A CLOSER LOOK

Dr. Michael Levy, *Attending Physician, Division of Pediatric Neurosurgery, Childrens Hospital Los Angeles, and Associate Professor of Neurosurgery, Keck School of Medicine, University of Southern California and Chairperson, American Academy of Pediatrics*

Closed head injuries, such as concussions, contusions, or cuts and lacerations, are caused by a blunt blow to the head. Closed head injuries during sports activities are common in children. No matter the cause, the best treatment is avoidance. Appropriate training of children on how to use sporting equipment, proper technique, and guidelines and instructions to both participants and spectators on the dangers is necessary.

Safety is a prime concern anytime children are involved in sports and games, especially for the head and eyes. Goggles should be worn for nearly all sports including baseball, basketball, karate, skiing, swimming, and racquetball. Good quality sports goggles can be purchased for less than twenty dollars and can be fitted with prescription lenses for those children who wear glasses.

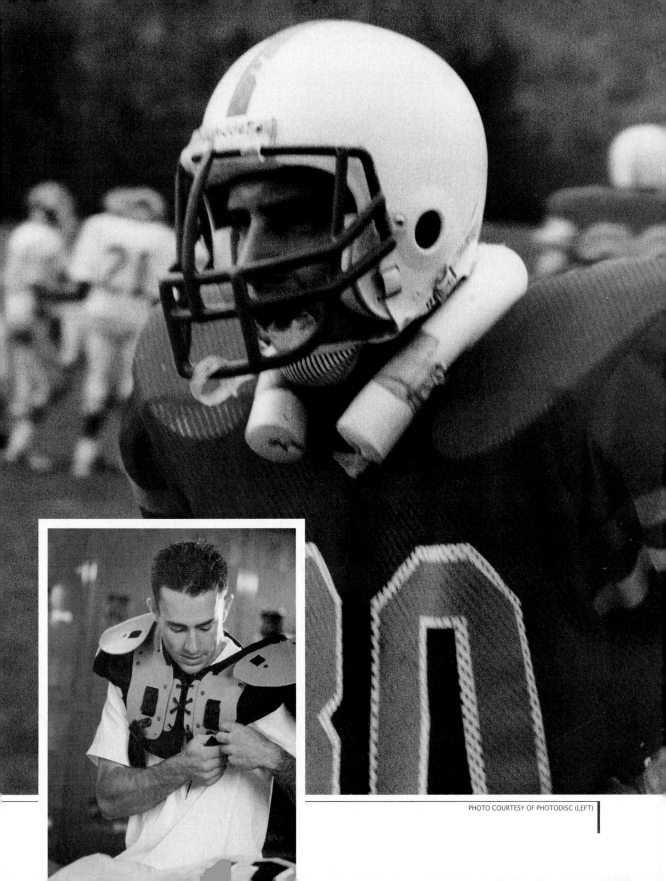

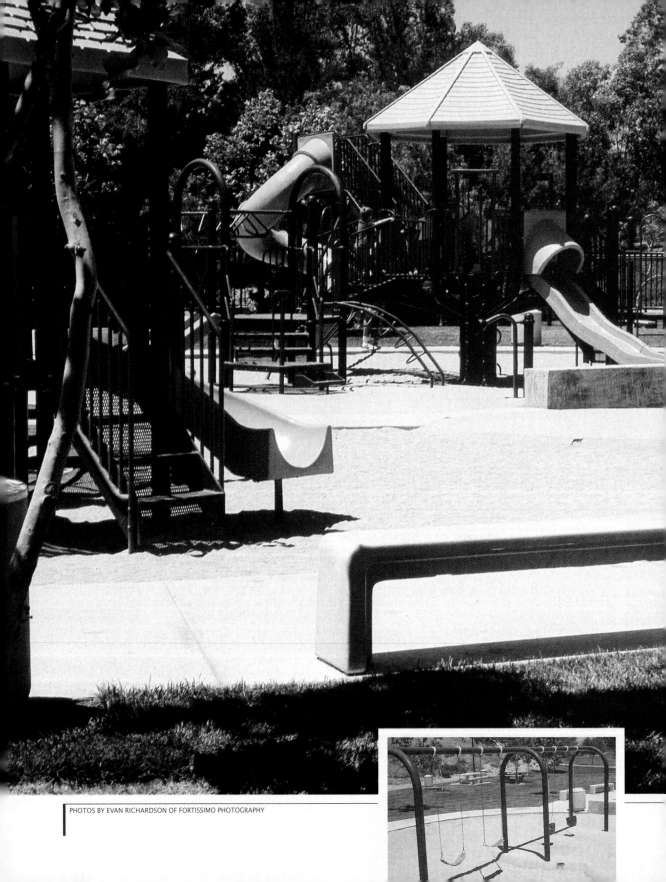

Playground Dangers

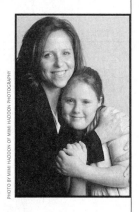

Most parents consider the playgrounds and parks where children play to be safe. However, even these child-friendly settings aren't as innocent as they may seem. As a parent, you need to watch everything your children do in these public places.

My daughter, Ellen, was nine years old and playing on a slide at the neighborhood playground when she lost her balance. She fell 8½ feet, hitting the ground. Her arm was broken in two places, requiring orthopedic surgery, the placement of two screws, and extensive physical therapy to repair the damage. Today, Ellen still has a scar. Now I always carefully examine any play equipment my children use—and I make sure that the right ground cover is present to cushion any falls that can't be avoided.

—*Ellen Sheehan*

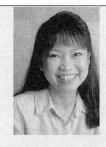

A CLOSER LOOK

Dr. Mary Ann Limbos, *Attending Physician, Division of General Pediatrics Childrens Hospital Los Angeles and Assistant Professor of Pediatrics, Keck School of Medicine, University of Southern California* Check playground equipment regularly for jagged edges or protrusions. See that hand-holds, seats, and footrests are fastened securely and platform areas have guardrails. Leave enough room between equipment so children don't crash into each other. Children should never play unattended. Make sure there's always adult supervision.

Keeping playground equipment safe requires choosing and maintaining the appropriate equipment for the age of children using the equipment. In particular, climbing equipment for children should be no higher than five feet for preschoolers and no higher than six feet for school-age children.

A Parent's quick checklist [11]

- Adult supervision is always present.
- Strings on clothes are removed.
- All children play on age-appropriate equipment.
- Falls to the ground are cushioned.
- All equipment is anchored to the ground and in good working order.

Safety checklists are available from the U.S. Consumer Product Safety Commission or the National Program for Playground Safety.

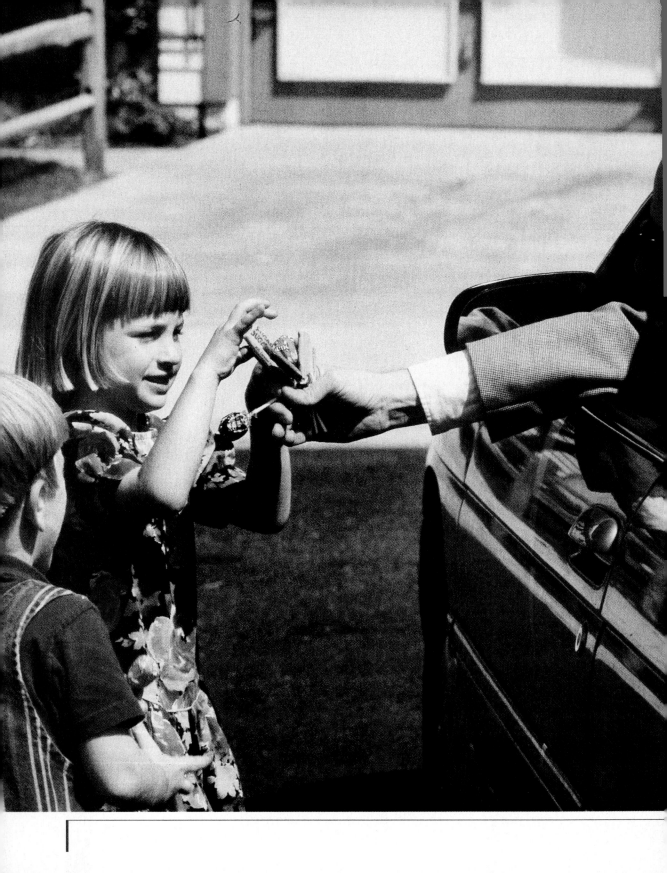

in-between

As parents, our children will not always be with us. Therefore, we must teach them to think about safety in every situation and to trust their instincts. If a situation feels unsafe, it usually is. Actively discuss safety with your child and encourage questions. To establish a dialogue on safety, communication must happen early and often. In addition, consider these guidelines when discussing safety with your child of any age:

- Communicate equal parts praise and guidance.
- Communicate capacity and independence.
- Use age-appropriate language and examples, such as the stories presented in this book.
- Be consistent with your limit setting and guidance. Be a role model; never practice "do as I say, not as I do," especially with safety equipment.
- Be sure to state to children that although certain behaviors are expected, they should be demonstrated not to please the parents, but for self-interest and personal safety.

Then when you are not with your child, the safety lessons learned will still be with your child.

—Efrain Garza Fuentes, Ed.D.
*Director, Patient & Family Services, Childrens
Hospital Los Angeles, and Voluntary Faculty
Member, Keck School of Medicine, University
of Southern California*

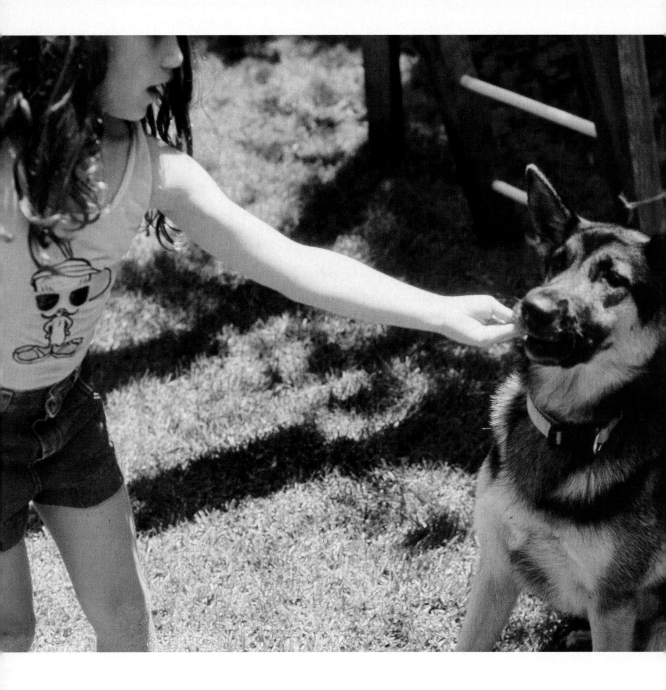

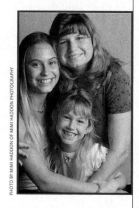

Show Caution Around Dogs

Children and animals seem to be a natural mix, especially when those animals are dogs. Because of this, dogs carry a special risk and as a parent you must be ever vigilant around them. One day, our family was visiting friends who had a dog. I assumed the dog was friendly because we knew the owners—something I will never do again. Our three-year-old daughter, Erin, started picking up one of the dog's plastic toys. The dog was instantly territorial. It bit her on the face, ripping through her lip and injuring her gums and teeth. There was a lot of blood and swelling. I applied ice while my husband drove us to the nearest hospital. There in the emergency room, Erin received stitches to close her wounds. She also needed to go to a dentist for follow-up care to repair the damage to her teeth and gums. The incidence was traumatic for all of us.

I can't stress enough the importance of exercising caution around any animal—particularly dogs. Tell your children not to play with a dog's toys or get near its food. Even when you think a situation is safe, it may not be.

—*Diane Grade*

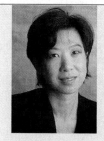

A CLOSER LOOK

Dr. Debra Don, *Attending Physician, Division of Otolaryngology, Childrens Hospital Los Angeles, and Assistant Professor, Pediatric Otolaryngology/Head and Neck Surgery, Keck School of Medicine, University of Southern California*

Dog bites are very common and can cause long-term disfigurement. Special care should always be taken when approaching a strange animal and children should be instructed to never touch an animal while it is eating. Finally, even dogs that you know can be dangerous if tired, hungry, or agitated.

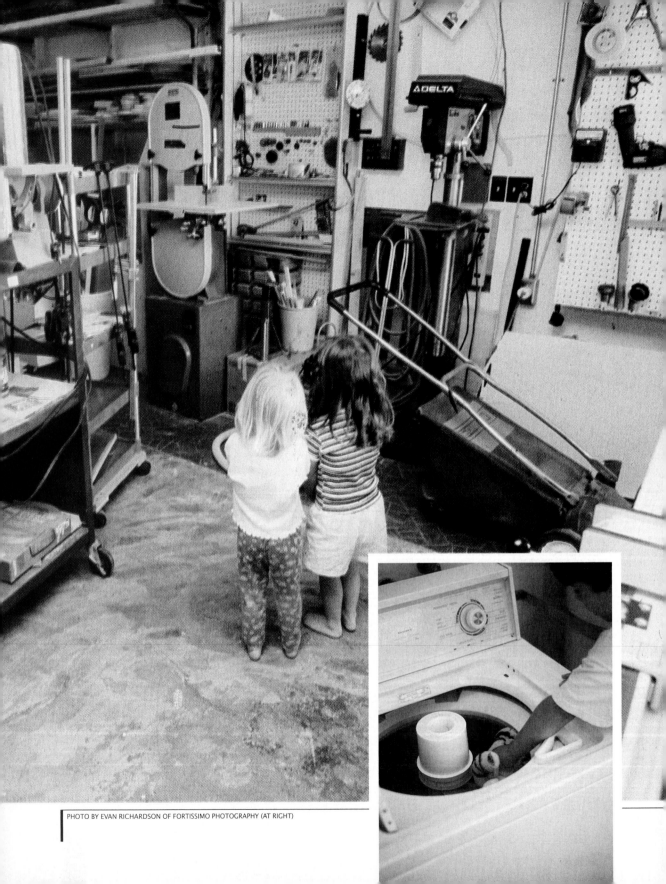

An Unsafe Washing Machine

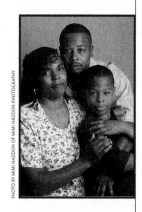

Parents are also consumers. In this dual role, we have a responsibility to demand safety in everyday household items. We found this out in the worst possible way. Our son, Malik, had his arm torn off when a washing machine in the laundromat did not turn off after the door was opened. When Malik's younger brother opened the washing machine door while it was running, Malik inserted his arm. Because the washing machine did not stop, Malik's arm was literally twisted from his elbow. Before the emergency response unit arrived, I had to force myself to reach into the washing machine and remove my son's arm. It was a good thing because the doctors were able to reattach the limb, even though they told us there was only a 25 percent chance of success. Malik has been through countless surgeries and still suffers nerve damage from the injury, but he has both his arms.

All of this could have been avoided, if a lock costing only eight dollars had been placed on the washing machine door. We would tell other parents to pay attention to all warning labels and be aware of their children's whereabouts. Never assume any item is safe, however ordinary.

—*Camille and Lamont Singletary*

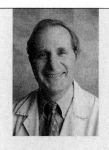

A CLOSER LOOK

Dr. John F. Reinisch, *Head, Division of Plastic Surgery, Childrens Hospital Los Angeles, and Associate Professor of Surgery, Keck School of Medicine, University of Southern California*
Life in a modern society is full of labor-saving devices that make daily chores quicker and less difficult. Although parents take many of our modern conveniences for granted, they hold a fascination for youngsters. Unfortunately, modern machinery and appliances do present a significant and constant health hazard for children. While some children have an innate sense of caution, many do not and are drawn to devices that make noise, move, or have lights. Car doors, exercise equipment, hot stoves and irons, escalators, and washing machines are commonly involved in injuries to arms, fingers, and legs in children. Parents need to be vigilant in all situations to avoid these types of injuries.

Caught in the Crossfire

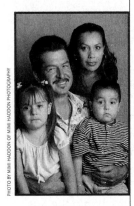

Gun violence seems to be everywhere. At the age of three, our son, Jesus, was shot in the back and remains paralyzed as a result. Jesus was outside with his father when the injury occurred. A wayward bullet struck him. The horror of seeing your child injured and then being rushed to the hospital cannot be adequately described in words. Jesus was in the hospital for many weeks and continues to receive rehabilitation in the hope he'll walk again. His injury has dramatically altered our home life and Jesus' life. He requires a wheelchair to move around and is unable to run and play with his friends. We urge all parents to practice gun safety. Ask other parents if they have guns in their homes and make sure that all guns are stored unloaded in a lock box. Don't be the next parent that has to see their child struck down in his or her prime.

—*Alma Gonzalez and Jesus Hernandez*

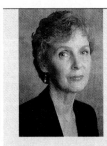

A CLOSER LOOK

Dr. Kathryn Anderson, *Surgeon-in-Chief, Childrens Hospital Los Angeles, and Division Chief, Pediatric Surgery and Professor of Surgery, Vice Chairman, Department of Surgery, Keck School of Medicine, University of Southern California*
Each year, 140 children under fifteen years of age die and 1,500 are injured in accidents involving guns [12]. A few simple steps can save your child's life:

1. At home, lock up all guns in a storage cabinet and use gun locks.
2. Store ammunition separately and never keep a loaded gun in the home.
3. Teach children to respect guns and that a gun is not a toy.
4. Ask the parents of your children's friends whether a gun is present in the home.

Dr. Mark Borchert, *Acting Division Head, Division of Ophalmology, Childrens Hospital Los Angeles and Associate Professor of Opthalmology and Neurology, Keck School of Medicine, University of Southern California*
Play violence such as rock throwing and "sword fighting" should be firmly prohibited. Finally, never allow your child to play with a youngster who has access to a BB gun. A BB gun has absolutely no value for hunting or protection, yet there is no more effective device for causing accidental blindness.

Also check out resources available from Children's Safety Network Resource Centers, including *Consumer Protection Approach to Firearm Safety, 1997,* and *Children, Adolescents, and Firearms* (1994).

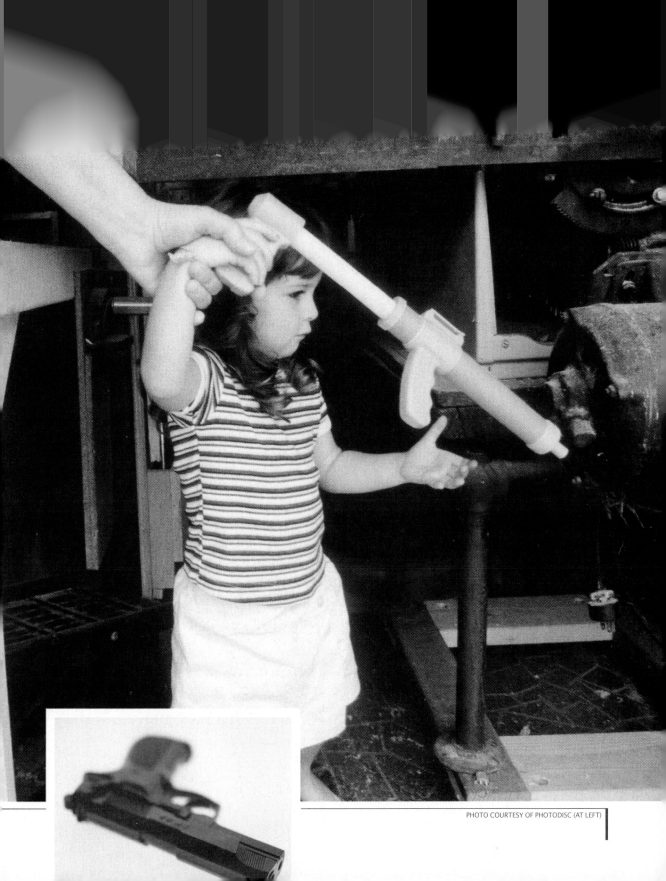

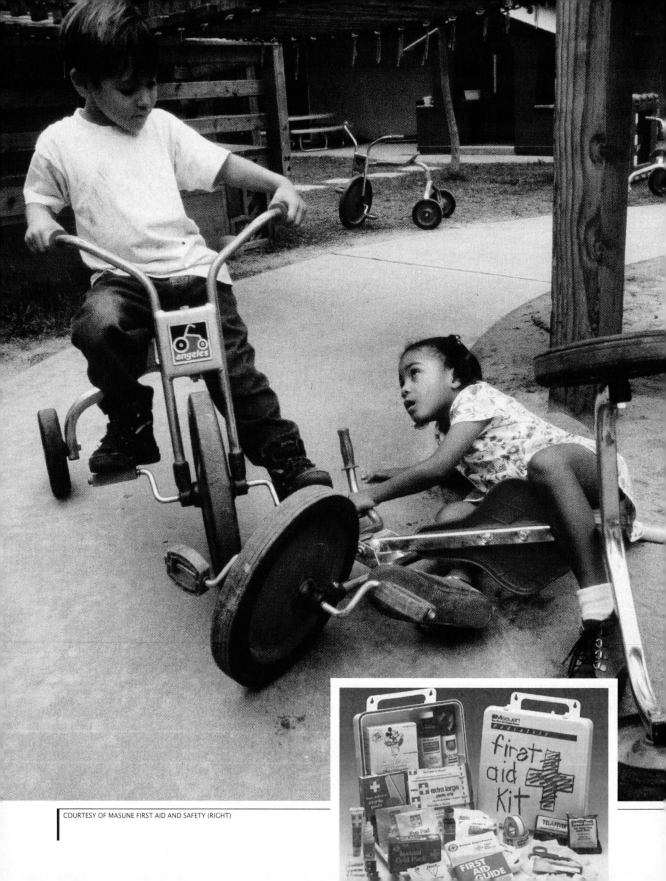

COURTESY OF MASUNE FIRST AID AND SAFETY (RIGHT)

Always Be Prepared

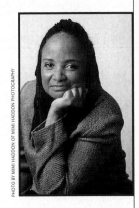

Knowing what to do and how to react in an emergency can make a big difference in the outcome. I learned this firsthand with my son, Adrian.

Adrian was six years old and had just started first grade. His teacher mentioned that he seemed to be having seizures and that we should watch him carefully. At the time, I was unsure of how to react and, looking back now, I know I should have sought help immediately. My son and I were on the way to the mall about three months later when he began to have a seizure in the car. I stopped the car and asked the first few people I saw for help but they only moved away. Finally, some nurses arrived and were able to calm me down. I then called 911. My son has not had a seizure since he was seven, but I would tell any parent whose child is prone to seizures to seek help immediately and not wait until an emergency arises. I was unprepared for the emergency and this could have resulted in a more serious injury to Adrian.

—*Patricia Henning*

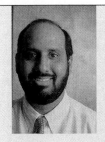

A CLOSER LOOK

Dr. Sajjad Yacoob, *Director, Undergraduate Medical Education, Childrens Hospital Los Angeles, and Attending Physician, Division of General Pediatrics, Childrens Hospital Los Angeles, and Assistant Professor of Pediatrics, Keck School of Medicine, University of Southern California*
Parents need to be prepared for emergencies by carrying a basic first aid kit, knowing the local emergency number, and if possible, carrying a cell phone. In addition, parents need to stay calm and be able to answer questions posed over the telephone about the condition of the child. Doing so will ensure that the proper treatment is delivered in a timely manner.

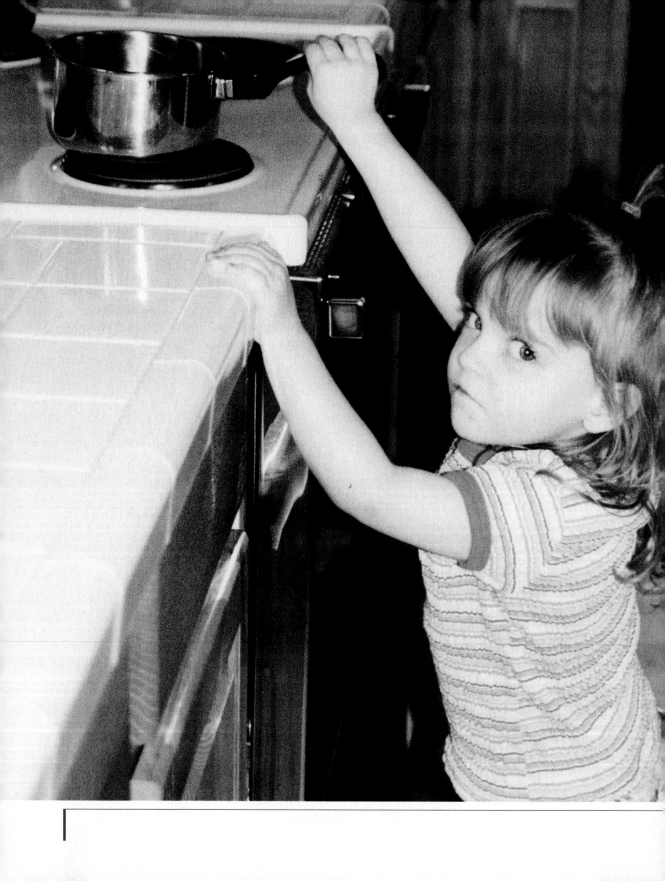

The Danger of Hanging Cords

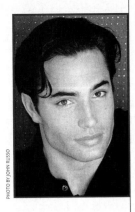

PHOTO BY JOHN RUSSO

When I was a little boy my mother was cooking in the kitchen with an electric frying pan. The cord to the frying pan was just long enough so that when it was hanging down the front of the cupboard, a curious little boy could grab it and pull. Fitting this description, I grabbed the cord and, to my mother's surprise and horror, pulled hard enough that the hot pan came flying at me, scalding grease and all. Fortunately, except for a few splatters of grease, I was not injured but I could have been seriously burned. We were lucky that day!

Parents need to pay close attention to hanging cords around the house, especially with curious little children exploring their surroundings. It is natural for a child to want to see what is going on in high places, so cords should be kept up out of reach—not hanging. The next curious child may not be so lucky when he pulls that cord. Who knows what the cord may be connected to? Quite possibly it will be connected to tragedy!

—Victor Webster

A CLOSER LOOK

Children's curiosity places them at a greater risk for burns since they are not always aware of potential dangers, especially in the kitchen. Never leave children in the kitchen, or other food preparation areas, without supervision. It is also important for you to assess your home and take precautions to prevent possible burns. For example, did you know that

scalding burns may be caused by—

- Boiling liquids or food on or off the stove
- Hot drinks or cereals that children like to drink, such as cocoa, or drinks left unattended, such as tea or coffee
- Steam from kettles, pans, hot cereal
- Hot water from the tap that is more than 120°F

contact burns may be caused by—

- A hot pan or pot on the stove
- Candles or candle wax left unattended
- Matches or lighters

electrical burns may be caused by—

- Touching a live wire
- Water contact with an electrical appliance, such as a toaster or electric hand mixer
- Sticking a foreign object into an electrical outlet

chemical burns may be caused by—

- Household chemicals, such as cleaners

(Adapted from *Safety, Nutrition, and Health in Early Education,* by Cathie Robertson, Delmar/ Thomson Learning)

The Shock of My Life

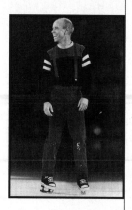

One of my favorite things to do when I was growing up was to sit and listen to my radio. One day I decided to rearrange my room and had to move the radio. When I went to plug it back in, I wasn't careful and my finger was in contact with the metal prong of the plug. I got the shock of my life!

To this day, I am *extremely* careful with anything involving electricity. As parents, you should make sure you supervise young children around appliances. Make sure children know how to use electrical appliances, or know to ask you or another adult for help if they don't, or your child could also have a very shocking experience!

—*Scott Hamilton*

A CLOSER LOOK

Electric shocks can be life-threatening, causing breathing to stop, severe burns, shock symptoms, and the heart to stop. Never touch a child, or anyone, who has received a serious electric shock until the source of electricity has been turned off or disconnected. Instead, use a dry, nonconductive object, such as a piece of wood, folded magazine, or rope to push or pull the child away from the source of the current. Also make sure you are standing on something dry, such as a board, when you are rescuing the child. Immediately unplug the cord, turn off the main breaker switch, or remove the fuse from the fuse box.

To treat a child who has received an electric shock:

1. Have someone call for emergency medical help while you remove the child from the source of the electric current.
2. If the child is pulseless and breathless, begin CPR.
3. Observe for signs of shock and burns, and treat as necessary.
4. Have the child transported to a medical facility as soon as possible.

(From *Health, Safety and Nutrition for the Young Child, 4th edition,* by Marotz, Cross & Rush, Delmar/Thomson Learning, © 1997.)

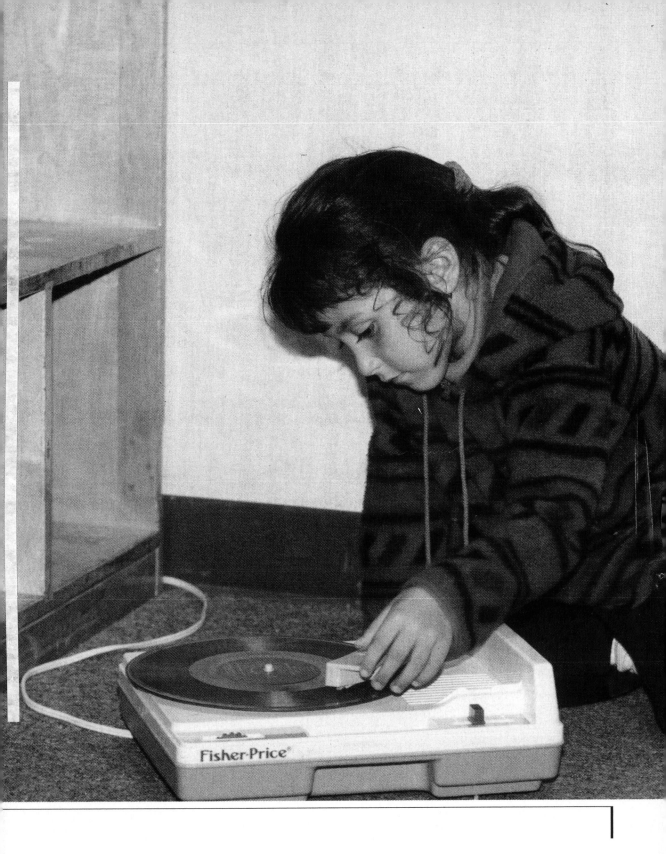

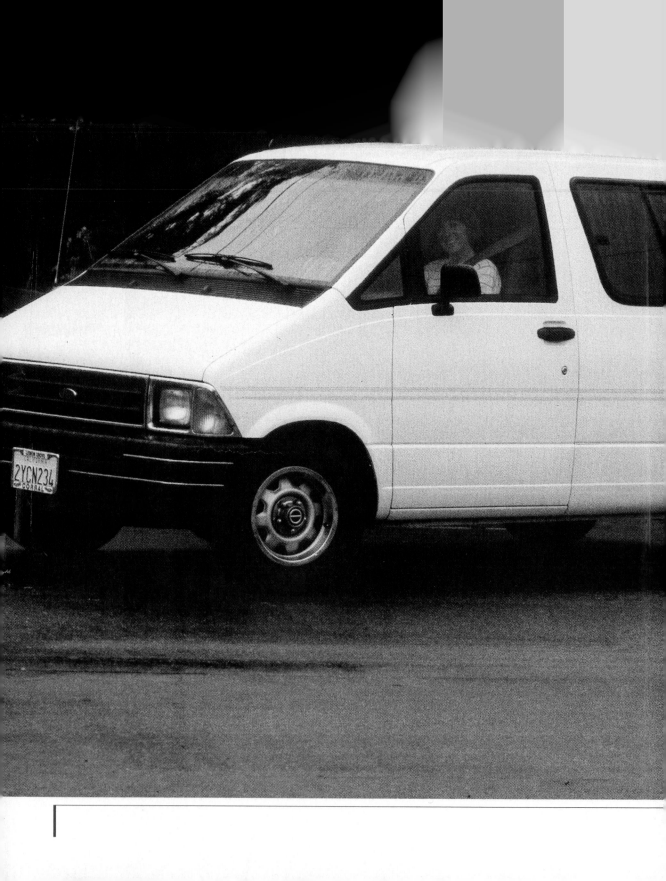

A Tree, a Steering Wheel, and Part of the Dashboard

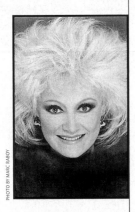

Never leave your car unlocked, even when it is in the garage. It is a terrible temptation to a kid of any age. Kids think what fun it would be to take the car out for a spin.

When I was nine, I started a car. I couldn't get it stopped, and became close friends with a tree, the steering wheel, and part of the dashboard. Because of my imprudence, I suffered half a century with an awful looking broken nose.

Cars are so easy to start now, even a dog can do it. My neighbor's dog, Spot, started their SUV and drove to Fresno before he was apprehended by the California Highway Patrol. He had picked up two hitchhikers and a nun—and they were all found singing "On the Road Again."

—Phyllis Diller

A CLOSER LOOK

The car can be a dangerous place for children, even when it's not in use. Always keep your car and trunk locked and, if possible, stored in a locked garage where it is not an inviting play area for your child. Also keep car keys well out of reach. Teach your child that the car is off-limits to them unless accompanied by you or another responsible adult.

Becoming locked inside of the trunk of a car, or "trunk entrapment," is a very serious problem. According to the National SAFE KIDS Campaign at least 260 people, 37 of whom were children ages 14 and under, have died in 229 incidents of trunk entrapment since 1970. The average age of children who have died in unintentional trunk entrapment incidents is 4 years old. Hyperthermia (heat stroke) or hyperthermia combined with asphyxiation is the most common cause associated with unintentional trunk entrapment deaths.

It is your job to—

- Teach kids not to play in or around cars.
- Always lock car doors and trunks, and keep the keys out of children's sight and reach.
- Supervise young children closely when they are around cars. Be especially careful when loading or unloading the trunk.
- Keep rear fold-down seats closed to help prevent kids from getting into the trunk from inside the car.

(From *Trunk Entrapment—the Facts*, the National SAFE KIDS Campaign, www.safekids.org)

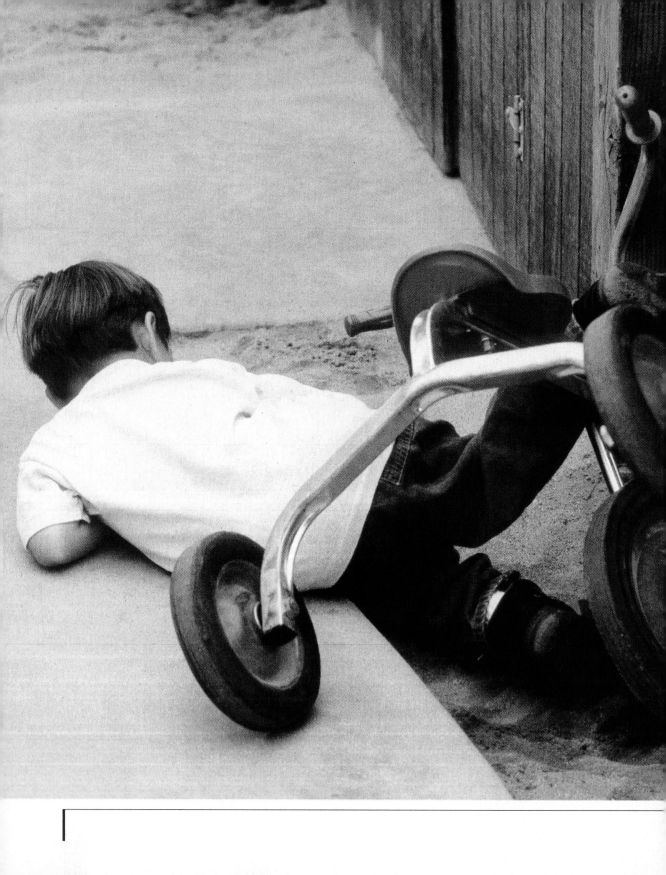

Protect Your Head

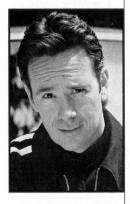

When I was eleven years old, I got a brand new BMX bike for my birthday. So the first thing I did was head down to the school-yard, without my helmet, and look for things to jump over. I thought the lunch table would be easy. But it turned out I was wrong. After the crash, it took thirty-six stitches to close up my face and head—and some very painful dental visits to replace my missing tooth.

Bike riding is great, but it is important to always stay within your limits. *Never* ride without a helmet. I drive race cars at 240 miles per hour, but I still will not get on my bike without a helmet. Believe me, concrete is hard! Always protect your head. Every time you ride.

—*Jimmy Vasser*

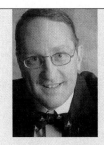

A CLOSER LOOK

Dr. Randall Wetzel, *Chairman, Department of Anesthesiology and Critical Care Medicine, the Anne O'M Wilson Professor of Critical Care Medicine, Director of Critical Care Medicine, Childrens Hospital Los Angeles, and Professor of Pediatrics and Anesthesiology, Keck School of Medicine, University of Southern California*

Head injuries suffered by children range from the trivial to severe injuries that result in permanent neurologic impairment, and even death. Seat belt and child safety laws have made a major impact on the incidence of childhood injuries and death from head trauma, but there are still thousands of children needlessly maimed and injured annually. This is particularly sad because preventive measures are available. Every year I see children who die, or are permanently injured from falling off skateboards, horses, and bicycles, or injure themselves on ski slopes or at baseball practice. All of these injuries could be prevented with the simple use of a properly fitted sports helmet.

Helmets have been mandated or recommended for a variety of sports and recreational activities including equestrian sports. Standards for helmets have been developed by the American Society for Testing and Materials, National Operating Committee on Standards for Athletic Equipment, Snell Memorial Foundation, and the American National Standards Institute. For specific information on the type of helmet required for your child's sports activity contact one of these organizations (see Appendix C).

A Hotel Disaster

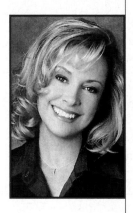

Please check and make sure things are nailed down in the hotel room when you are traveling with children.

I was with my two-year-old daughter in New York City. There was a TV in our room that was sitting, unattached, on top of a table. The table was too light for the TV, and the bottom rollers were unstable. When my daughter stepped on the lower shelf to reach up to the set, the eighty-pound TV came down on her chest.

They closed down the Verrazano Bridge to get her to the emergency room. Blood was pouring out of her ear, and she was unconscious for ten minutes. If the New York Police had not been so great (and if the in-house detective had not been involved) I do not know what would have happened.

At the hospital, the nuns rang the bells, and everybody prayed. After two days and nights, the tests came back fine. I thanked the nun, and started to tell her that I prayed that there would be no future damage, but she stopped me before I finished the sentence and said, "Accept the miracle!"

—Catherine Hicks

A CLOSER LOOK

Young children are curious and eager to explore every inch of your hotel or motel room, usually while you are on the phone or otherwise preoccupied with the details of your trip. As a parent, it is your job to check things out thoroughly first to create a safe environment for your children.

Look around the room to see what small objects, such as matchbooks, pens, pen caps, or coins, have been left lying in reach of children and place them out of reach. Don't forget to look inside dresser and desk drawers, inside closets, and under the bed and furniture. Check the draperies or other window coverings for potentially hazardous pull cords and lift them out of reach. Become familiar with the locking mechanism on the window; is there a safety guard in place, or can your children fit through the opening? If yes, ask the hotel management if they can supply a window guard, or consider moving to another room or hotel.

Look to see if electrical cords from lamps and other appliances are hanging low enough for toddlers to chew, pull, or trip on. Carry safety caps for wall outlets with you in case the hotel does not supply them. Once inside, keep all hotel doors and windows locked, even when everyone is in the room, and instruct children to never open the door for anyone who is unknown to them, even if the person claims to be from room service. Finally, learn the location of all fire exits and elevators by studying the hotel floor plan, and take a walk with your children to physically locate them.

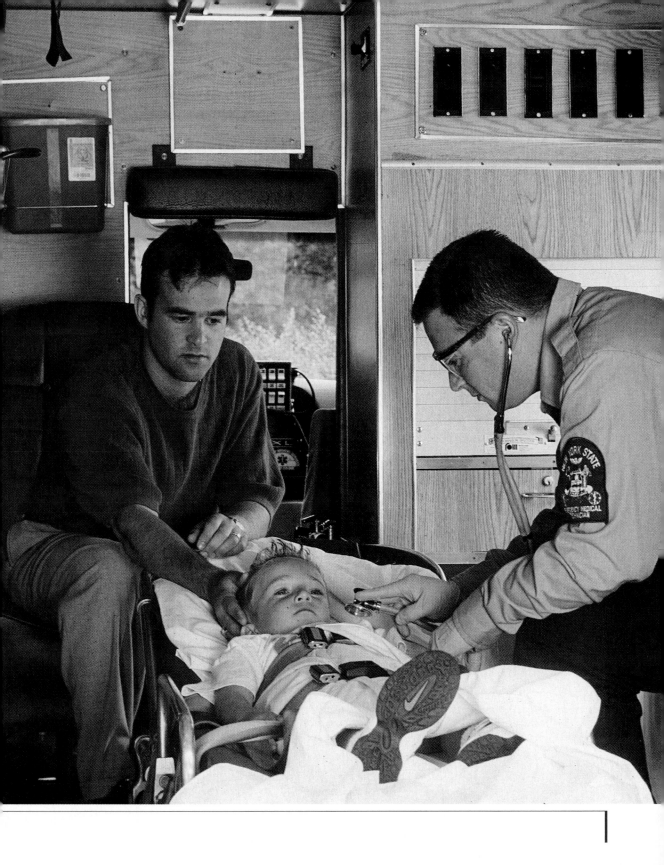

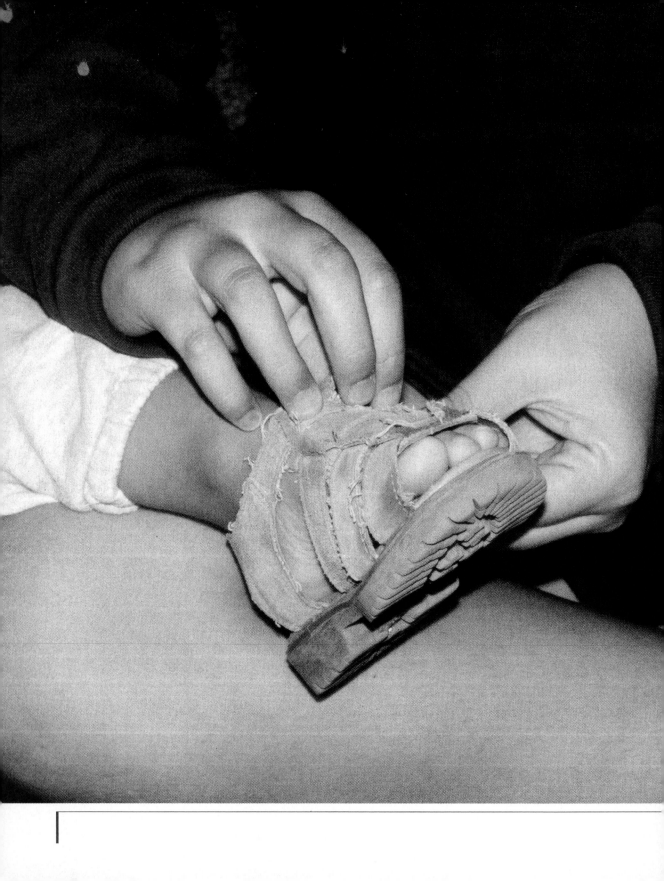

Protect Your Feet

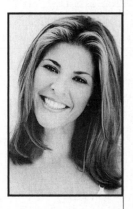

My mom always warned me to wear shoes when heading for the outdoors, but I did not always listen. One day when I was four years old, I ran outside to play hide-and-seek with some friends. I was confident that I would be just fine without something on my feet. As I ran along the side of the house to the perfect hiding spot, I stepped on a board with a nail in it. The nail went right through my foot, sticking up all the way to the other side. Oh, how I have never forgotten the pain of them pulling that nail out . . . the doctor's prickly tetanus shot . . . and all the stitches that followed!

So from that awful experience, I have learned: "When heading for the street, always protect your precious feet!"

—*Rita Sever*

A CLOSER LOOK

Children should be encouraged to wear shoes, sneakers, sandals or other foot protection while walking or playing outdoors. If this is not possible in all areas, such as around a swimming pool, make sure surfaces are safe and free of sharp stones, debris, small toys, or other items that might cause lacerations or tripping. Also take care to properly dispose of feces from pets.

If your child's foot has been injured you will need to take a few precautions to ensure proper healing after the initial medical treatment to clean and treat the injury. For example:

- Keep the injured foot clean and dry at all times
- Make sure your child wears socks until the wound is healed, but avoid 100% cotton socks since they will stay wet
- Check the wound for signs of infection, such as redness around site, swelling, or discharge and seek medical attention

Finally, are your children up-to-date on all necessary immunizations? The Td (tetanus and diphtheria toxoids) is recommended for children 11 to 12 years of age and subsequent Td boosters are recommended every 10 years. Check with your children's pediatrician each time you visit them to make sure their immunizations are current. Additional information on immunization and recommended schedules may be found on the American Academy of Pediatrics website at www.aap.org.

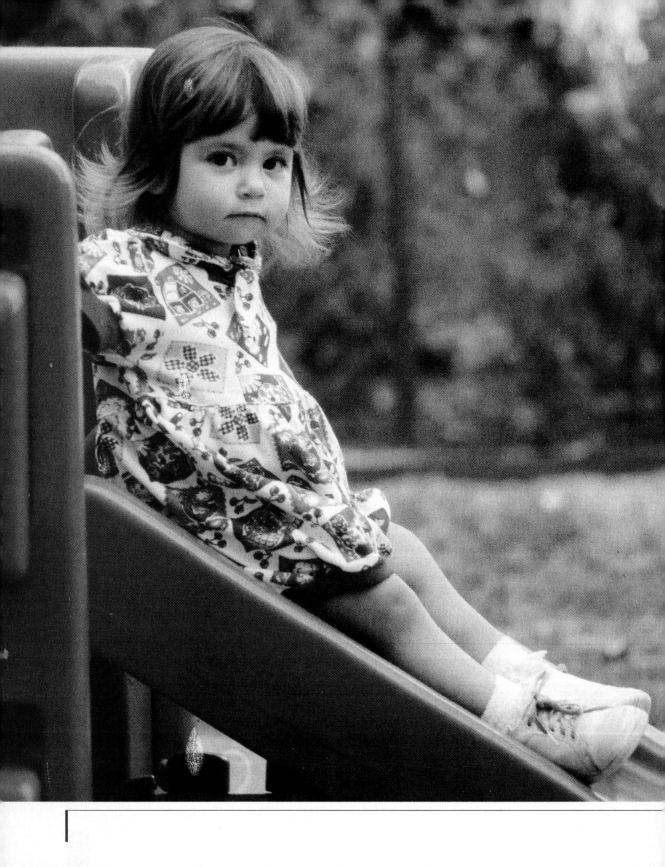

lessons learned

The information in this section is provided not to scare parents, but rather to reinforce the importance of injury prevention. Parents often see injuries to children as unavoidable. Although every child will suffer minor scrapes and bruises, no child should have to suffer serious injury from a preventable event. Therefore, when reading this information, think about what you can do *today* to decrease risk of injury to the children entrusted to your care, whether you are a parent, grandparent, or caretaker.

Please also refer to the resources and guidelines included in the Appendices at the end of the book. Appendix D provides a summary of quick tips you can use based on the age of your child. Take the time to review this information and choose at least one tip to implement today.

Severe Injuries

Patient and Family Care Services, Childrens Hospital Los Angeles

Everyone deals with stress differently, however, the stress associated with the severe injury of a child is profoundly unique. As such, it deserves specific discussion because of the ripple effect of this stress on the entire family unit. Therefore, this chapter will look at the effects of a severe injury on the family unit and also discuss the effects of this stress.

It has been said that "if a disease were killing our children in the proportions that accidents are, people would be outraged and demand that this killer be stopped" (C. Everett Koop, M.D., Sc.D., former Surgeon General, National SAFE KIDS Campaign). Recent advances in the prehospital setting, emergency room, operating room, and intensive care units of organized pediatric trauma centers have resulted in improved survival in those with serious multisystem injuries. Nevertheless, as the delivery of pediatric trauma care has improved, a new problem has come into focus— critically injured children survivors and their families make up a group with significant long-term care issues that have only recently been identified (4).

The impact of a severe injury or death of a child on a family can be affected by a variety of factors including the severity of the injury, the social environment (e.g., other family stressors), and the availability of resources [13(p658)]. In addition to concerns about the child's recovery, the family is also concerned about interactions with other family members, siblings, and grandparents [13(p658)]. Another practical burden is the financial hardship that is often faced by families with a child who has been severely injured. We will examine the stressors in chronological order as they occur in realtime when a child is severely injured.

Immediate Stress Following the Injury

For most parents, the immediate stress is focused on ensuring that the child is receiving appropriate care, not suffering any pain, and reassuring the child that mom or dad is there if needed. There are feelings of helplessness and loss of power, and many parents are overwhelmed by feelings of inadequacy and guilt [14(p69)]. Many will begin to search for explanations or ask themselves, "How could I let this happen to my child?" [14(p69)].

Once the child is out of immediate danger and has reached the rehabilitation stage, most parents begin to focus on recovery and its expectations. This search for answers is also stressful because parents often deny the extent or permanence of likely disabilities [15(p663)]. Denial may be a coping mechanism for some parents, but it can lead to profound sadness and parents may begin to experience what some have called "partial death" and "mobile mourning" [15(p663)]. "Their child is alive but is not the child they knew before the injury" [15(p663)]. The parents may grieve at the time of the injury, but they tend to grieve over and over again [15(p663)]. Children whose injuries are not as severe often suffer a unique sort of stress associated with comparisons of before and after the injury and changes in level and ability. Sometimes they are termed "almosters"—they can almost learn, play, etc., like they used to [15(p663)]. For the parents of a severely injured child a phenomenon called the "Lazarus phenomenon" may occur, in which the parents withdraw from the child [17(p197)]. The parents prepare for the child's death only to have the child live day after day, week after week [17(p1977)]. The act of the child living begins a cycle of guilt by the parent, who may unconsciously wish his or her child to die, but feels guilty for thinking such thoughts. This leads to sadness, anger, and anxiety that are not likely to decrease over time. Recent studies [18] point to ongoing physical disabilities that limit the child's participation in normal activities and make it difficult to integrate the injured child back into the home setting.

The Stress of Returning Home

The next step in the recovery process is the stress of returning home. For the parent of a child who has suffered a severe injury, the stress can be enormous. The family may need to deal with finding alternative care, school accommodations, and in some cases home placement for a child. One parent may be forced to give up a job or travel great distances to ensure adequate medical care and education for the child [15(p 664)]. Coping resources will be taxed because of the need to accommodate a wide variety of tasks. In addition to the stress of caring for a severely injured child, there is the financial strain associated with medical and legal costs, as well as ongoing rehabilitation and costs related to modifying the home environment [15(p664)]. Other stress factors include the time-consuming and difficult task of securing assistance such as Social Security. Mothers, in particular, suffer from increased stress and higher rates of depression because the primary task of raising a severely injured child often falls to them [20(pp682–685)].

Stress on Other Family Members

Beyond the stress to the parent of a severely injured child, there is the stress suffered by other members of the family unit including brothers and sisters, grandparents, and other caretakers. This may result in other family members attempting to secure additional attention while feeling guilty about asking for the attention [15,(p664)]. Studies have also found that siblings of disabled children are more aggressive, which can affect their ability to learn effectively in a school setting, and that over time the problems do not reduce significantly [16(pp1042–44)]. These effects eventually lead to social isolation that can interfere with normal peer and adolescent relationships and may continue to plague the siblings into young adulthood [16(p1045)]. Additional stress may occur as a result of unwanted advice from neighbors and the community, including schools which are often poorly prepared to deal with a child's special needs [21(p189)].

Long-term Effects of Stress

The stress of external forces are tremendous, but there also is stress from internal forces, such as separation, divorce, and the rare return of an estranged parent. Studies show that at the end of the first year after an injury the composition of the family changes in 40 percent of families studied [22].

As the severely injured child is reintegrated into the family unit, the level of stress may decrease but will never go away completely. The parent must accept that their child has changed forever and they must shift expectations, give up dreams and sometimes accept the fact of a lifetime of dependency [15(p664)]. Therefore, it is critical that any parent of a severely injured child reach out and request help as needed. This will help lower the level of stress and avoid some of the unintended consequences of that stress.

Effects on the Injured Child

Immediately following a severe injury the child may be totally unaware of any loss in abilities, but as the child progresses a realization of the loss will occur. Initially, the child may suffer from fear, anxiety, terror, and depression [19(p154)]. Eventually, the child will begin to develop coping techniques and to reshape their body image to better fit current realities [19(p154)]. However, the extent of recovery is often directly linked to the strength of the family unit at a time when the family unit is stretched thin [21(p191)]. Therefore, the newly disabled child often becomes depressed and withdraws [21(p192)]. In some cases, the withdrawal leads to social maladjustment and antisocial behavior, which in turn leads to difficulty in school and other social settings [22(p108)].

Isolation not only affects the child, it also affects the family. The family often becomes less active because of the difficulty in transporting and caring for a child outside the home. This too becomes a self-defeating cycle and leads to increased levels of depression and anxiety.

Conclusion

Traumatic injuries to children have far-reaching consequences that extend beyond the bruises, scars, and physical disabilities that result from the injury itself. These effects are often known as the "hidden morbidity" in pediatric trauma, or a diseased state that manifests itself not only as physical disability but also as changes in cognition, personality, and behavior, and as family stress [4]. As the stories in this book have shown, these injuries are preventable in most cases by following steps to avoid them, including using recommended safety equipment and following common sense precautions.

Death

More than 20,000 children and young adults will die this year as a result of injury [3]. Many of the stresses related to the death of a child are unique to the individual family and, consequently, require a separate discussion. However, the death of a child does create some statistically measurable effects on parents, including the breakup of the existing marriage or relationship, an increased incidence of maternal smoking during the next pregnancy, and eventually the adjustment of family size to compensate for the loss [23(p946)]. Recent data indicate that the divorce rate for parents of a deceased child is about 12 percent; of which one in four couples report that the death of their child contributed to the divorce [28].

Beyond divorce and direct stress on the marriage and relationship, the sudden death of a child is considered a more drastic event than a death following chronic illness [24(p281)]. As a result, the outcome for the family unit can be more extreme. Parents suffer intense grief, depression, as well as anger and guilt with accompanying despair and alienation [25(p310)]. Parental suffering often manifests in negative behavior such as drinking and sleeping problems [26(p77)]. Parents also report physical symptoms including high blood pressure, colds, influenza, arthritis, infections, chest pain, and skin allergies [27(p572)]. The unnatural occurrence of a child's death complicates the normal grieving process because parents do not expect to outlive their children [27(pg. 572)]. Consequently, parents often report that they never truly recover [27(p572)].

Most parents find out about the death of their child from an injury at the hospital or trauma center, and are told of the death by the attending physician and/or trained social worker. Initially, parents express disbelief and often request to see the child [27]. The parents will hold the child and begin to understand the permanence of the child's state. It is at this time that a parent will start to question why, and may begin to lay blame and focus on regrets [27]. Parents must also face the task of telling other family members, other children, and friends, as well as the reactions of those individuals.

Siblings also suffer immense grief at the loss and may find it difficult to express their feelings because of not wanting to "make their parents cry." In addition, many studies have shown that siblings experience guilt, especially very young children who do not understand cause-and-effect relationships [28]. Other children may believe that the death of a sibling is a form of punishment [28]. The intense emotions experienced by siblings can be very difficult for a parent to deal with because they are also dealing with their own grief; this can lead to both the child and the parent not completing the grieving process [28].

The circle of grief also includes grandparents, caretakers, and friends. Grandparents often experience a double grief—sorrow for their child who is suffering and sorrow over their own loss of a grandchild. This can lead to a grandparent's efforts being interpreted as taking control or overstepping their boundaries and resentment between the parent and grandparent [29].

Caretakers and friends also suffer, especially if the child was older and had an established network of close friends. Adolescent friends may become angry or preoccupied with death [30]. Although these groups traditionally fare much better than parents, it does not mean that their feelings of loss are easily overcome.

After the funeral, the process of grieving continues. There is no set time for completion of the grieving process, which is unique for each parent and family unit. Although parents begin to understand that the child will never return, they often say that they are changed forever.

Pediatric Trauma: Prevention Strategies

Steven Stylianos, M.D.
Associate Professor of Clinical Surgery and Pediatrics at Columbia University College of Physicians and Surgeons, Director, Regional Pediatric Trauma Program Childrens' Hospital of New York, and Chairman, Trauma Committee, American Pediatric Surgical Association.

Injury is the most significant threat to the health of children in the United States and the leading cause of death after the first year of life. Each year, nearly 13 million children from birth to fourteen years of age visit emergency rooms in the United States; 360,000 are hospitalized; 8,000 die; and a significant number are left with a permanent disability (see Table 1) [42,58]. The most important step in preventing injuries is overcoming a sense of fatalism, that injuries are "accidents" or random events that cannot be predicted. Fatalism holds that events are fixed for all time in such a manner that individuals, be they lay persons or professionals, are powerless to change them [47].

TABLE 1	Leading Causes of Pediatric Trauma Deaths
Traffic-related	56%
Homicide	17%
Drowning	11%
Burns/inhalation	7%
Falls and other	10%

Injury is a disease that depends on the principles of epidemiology, engineering, biomechanics, and health education for prevention (see Table 2). The concept of an "accident-prone child" shifts attention away from potential interventions, through products or the environment. The tremendous toll injuries take on children and their families can only be reduced by coupling effective prevention and intervention strategies with improvements in the access to and delivery of pediatric trauma care [45,4].

TABLE 2	Prevention Strategies for Common Pediatric Injuries
Type of Injury	**Intervention**
Motor vehicle accident, occupant	Child car seat / Seat belt
Motor vehicle accident, pedestrian	School-based safety program
Bicycle	Helmet
Drowning	Pool fencing
Burn	Smoke detector / Tap water regulator / Flammable Fabric Act
Fall	Window guard
Poisoning	Preventive Packaging Act
Homicide	Handgun legislation / Crisis resolution counseling

Injuries are not random events but occur in predictable patterns based in part on age, gender, time of day, and season of the year. Haddon proposed a multifaceted, multidisciplinary approach to lessen the likelihood of childhood injury nearly two decades ago (see Table 3), a model applicable to our clinical practice today [43,44]. The Haddon matrix, a model for understanding injuries, divides an injury occurrence into three phases (see Table 4). Within each phase are opportunities to prevent injuries and lessen their impact.

TABLE 3	Ten Intervention Strategies to Lessen the Likelihood of Injury or to Minimize the Consequence on Injury [43]

1. Prevent the creation or marshaling of the hazard.
   Example: Prevent the manufacture of handguns.
2. Reduce the amount of the hazard.
   Example: Package children's medicines in nonlethal quantities.
3. Prevent the inappropriate release of an existing hazard.
   Example: Teach children to swim.

(continued)

TABLE 3 (*continued*)

4. Modify the release or spatial distribution of the hazard.
   Example: Require the use of child safety seats for young children.
5. Separate the hazard from the child in time or space.
   Example: Provide bicycle paths away from automobile traffic.
6. Physically separate the hazard from the child.
   Example: Use plastic covers for electric outlets.
7. Modify the structure of the hazard.
   Example: Surround playground equipment with wood chips rather than concrete.
8. Increase the child's resistance to the hazard.
   Example: Increase children's musculoskeletal strength through exercise and fitness programs.
9. Begin to counter damage already done.
   Example: Train paramedics to treat childhood injuries.
10. Stabilize, repair, and rehabilitate the injured child.
    Example: Establish regional pediatric trauma centers and rehabilitation facilities.

TABLE 4 **The Haddon Matrix: Understanding Injury Causation**

	Pre-event	Event	Post-event
Host	Alcohol abuse	Seat belt use	Trauma service
	Age	Osteoporosis	Rehab care
	Cognitive impairment	Age	
Vector	Anti-lock brakes	Air bag	Fuel system
	Travel speed	Side impact protection	integrity
Physical Environment	Road surface	Guard rails	EMS system
	Highway design	Breakaway poles	
	Lighting		
Social Environment	DWI laws	Car design laws	Job retraining
	Seat belt laws		EMS support

Methods aimed at reducing childhood injury are described as active or passive. Active intervention requires a behavior change such as wearing a seat belt, while passive intervention requires little action on the part of the individual being protected, for example, an automobile air bag. Active interventions are more likely to be effective if the actions required are simple, inexpensive, and not repetitive. Passive interventions, while more effective, cannot be applied to all types of injury risk. To the extent that passive intervention is limited, we must depend on altering the behaviors that put our children at risk. Efforts to persuade individuals, particularly parents, to change their behaviors have constituted the greater part of injury control efforts in this country. In contrast, the most successful injury prevention programs are those involving product design, which protect all individuals regardless of cooperation or level of skill. Active and passive interventions can be combined in specifically targeted programs such as reducing teenaged driver collisions (see Table 5). Legislation and regulation at the national, state, and local levels, such as requiring safety seats and bicycle helmets, have been effective in reducing many types of childhood injury.

TABLE 5	**Active and Passive Strategies Aimed at Reducing Teenaged Driving Collisions**
Strategy	*Type*
Increasing the age of licensure	Passive
Eliminating driver education classes that enable drivers to become licensed at younger ages	Passive
Increasing the legal drinking age	Passive
Enacting night time driving curfews	Active and passive
Promoting the use of safety belts	Active
Stricter penalties for DWI	Passive

Successful injury prevention programs should incorporate the four *E*s: *E*ngineering of products and environments; *E*nactment (and enforcement) of legislation or regulations to promote safety; *E*ducation of children, caregivers, health-care professionals, and legislators; and *E*valuation of the efficacy of specific interventions.

Motor Vehicle Accidents

Motor vehicle accidents (MVA) and traffic-related injuries are the leading cause of traumatic death to children and adolescents, accounting for 56 percent of injury fatalities [41,59]. These injuries can occur at speeds as low as twenty-five to thirty miles per hour and the severity of injury often reflects the type of passenger restraint used. Patterns of injury based on age, seat location, and type of restraint reveal sharp contrasts in pediatric injury patterns based on the use or nonuse of seat belts [32,35,54]. The severity of injuries, including the severity of Glasgow Outcome Score (see Table 6), and length of hospital stays are significantly increased for children who are not properly restrained in motor vehicles. The subject of car restraints for infants and children has attracted a great deal of attention by the public and automotive industry. Seat belts and car seats undeniably save lives if used properly. However, the issues of proper design and compliance are not entirely solved. Recent legislation has made three-point restraints standard in the rear seats of American-made automobiles which may decrease the incidence of the "seat belt syndrome" in children [49].

TABLE 6	**Glasgow Outcome Scale**

1 = death

2 = persistent vegetative state

3 = severe disability (requires assistance with activities of daily living)

4 = moderate disability (independent, but disabled)

5 = mild or no disability (capacity to resume normal occupational and social activities)

The National Highway Traffic Safety Administration estimates that 500 deaths and 53,000 injuries could be prevented each year with proper use of child safety seats and if compliance with existing state law was 100 percent. Encouraging statistics from Michigan and California support this position. The enactment of child safety seat legislation illustrates the joint effectiveness of legislation and education (passive and active strategies) in reducing the risk of childhood injury [59].

However, the legislation means nothing if every parent does not take the time to properly secure their own child. This means using the recommended infant seat, car seat, or booster until the child is eight, and securing every child who is older than eight with a seat belt.

Bicycle Injuries

Bicycle injuries to children and adolescents result in more than 400,000 emergency room visits and 600 deaths annually. Nearly 25 percent of all significant brain injury to children 14 years old or younger are bicycle-related. The most successful efforts to reduce injury among pediatric bicyclists focus upon increasing helmet use [34,35,39].

A study from Seattle, Washington, showed a reduction of head and central nervous system injury by 85 percent with proper helmet usage [55]. The Seattle program relied on physician handouts, public service announcements, manufacturer and retailer discounts, and recruitment of local sports figures as spokespersons.

In Ontario, a review of coroner's records during a five-year period identified 81 children who died from bicycle injuries [53]. Head injury contributed to 89 percent of the deaths; none of the 81 victims were wearing a helmet. Grassroots efforts to distribute educational materials that increase public awareness of the importance of bicycle helmets will remain a critical component in attempts to decrease the morbidity of these preventable injuries.

Although many publicity campaigns have focused on bicycle safety, it is important to remember that safety equipment needs to be used whenever a child is using a ride-on toy, including skateboards, in-line skates, motorized scooters, tricycles, and motorized go-carts. In addition, parents must carefully read the instructions included with the ride-on toy, abide by age guidelines, and provide adult supervision at all times.

Pedestrian Injury

Pedestrian injury results in nearly 2,000 deaths of children between the ages of one to 14 years annually. Unfortunately, there are no simple solutions to this complex problem and no single intervention capable of producing large and uniform reductions in injury. School-based programs focused on specific age groups have been the most effective programs to date [37,38,52]. These programs aim to improve the street-crossing skills of children with the use of animated films, posters, public service announcements, and training sessions in real traffic situations or simulations.

Pedestrian injuries are best avoided by parents acting as role models. Every parent should follow traffic signals and teach their children to do the same. In addition, everyone can help reduce this problem by not running red lights, following the posted speed limits, and carefully following traffic signs that designate school zones and play areas.

Drownings

Drowning ranks second only to MVAs as the most common cause of "accidental" death in children [46]. More than 2,000 children drown each year in the United States [57]. The primary strategy to prevent drownings and near drownings in residential swimming pools is use of latch-gate fences that separate the pool from the house and yard. Australian studies have described a four-fold decrease in residential drownings with strict pool fencing regulations [50]. Proper pool fencing, pool covers, and CPR training for all pool owners can prevent up to 90 percent of all residential drownings. A telephone at poolside can eliminate a potential distraction of a parent while a toddler is near the water, as long as the telephone itself does not become a distraction.

Adult supervision is absolutely necessary whenever children are in and around water. Parents and caretakers must also ensure that proper safety equipment such as life preservers are used and a fence is installed. Finally, never rely on a child to supervise him or herself.

Burns

Approximately 1,200 children under the age of 15 die in residential house fires annually; more than half of them are under five years old. Half of these house fires are started by cigarettes. Smoke inhalation poses as great a risk to infants and children as the fire itself. With limited mobility, infants and toddlers may be away from the flames but succumb to inhaled smoke.

Smoke detectors have been estimated to reduce the likelihood of death in a house fire by 85 percent. Strategies to combat this problem include smoke detector programs in low-income neighborhoods, development of plans for a family escape route, and installation of heat-activated sprinkler systems [40,48].

An area where focused intervention has made a significant impact in reducing burn injuries is in the materials of children's clothing. In 1967 the federal Flammable Fabrics Act was passed requiring children's sleepwear to be flame-retardant [51]. Clothing ignition burns now account for only a small percentage of burns in children as a result of this legislation. It is distressing to note recent pressures on the Consumer Product Safety Commission to relax standards for children's clothing.

Each year over 35,000 children sustain scald burns. Another example of product modification resulting in substantial reduction of injury involves water heater temperature limits. Bath and tap water scalds increase markedly as temperatures rise above 130 degrees Fahrenheit. Legislation in the State of Washington was passed in 1983 requiring new water heaters to be preset at 120 degrees Fahrenheit, a temperature at which dishwashers and washing machines still operate effectively. As a result of the law and a public education campaign, 77 percent of homes had tap water temperatures below 130 degrees as compared to 20 percent 10 years earlier [51]. The number of tap water scald victims admitted to the hospital was decreased by half during this period.

Caretakers and parents should always check the temperature of water with an elbow before placing a child in water, even if the water was checked originally. The temperature can change as water is added. Finally, always place pots on the back burners of a stove and teach your child that the oven is hot. This lesson can start as soon as the child begins to move around.

Poisonings

The reduction of poisoning deaths among young children over the past quarter-century represents the epitome of successful injury control. Between 1970 and 1985, the number of poisoning deaths among children younger than five years decreased by 75 percent [58]. The Poison Preventive Packaging Act of 1970 required childproof closures on 16 categories of medications and toxic household agents [51,56]. This legislation combined with dose limits per package, regional poison control centers, and pediatrician counseling continues to protect children.

To prevent poisonings, parents need to keep poisons out of reach by locking cabinets and placing the poisons in childproof containers.

Falls

Falls from heights are a major cause of traumatic death and serious disability in urban children. Two decades ago, falls accounted for 12 percent of all unintentional traumatic deaths of children in New York City [33]. In 1972, The New York City Department of Health developed a health education program, Children Can't Fly. Inexpensive window guards were obtained and installed on apartment windows of the second floor and above, and the New York City Health Code was revised in 1976 to require guards on all windows of apartments in which a child under the age of 11 resided. Since then there has been a 96 percent decrease in falls through windows.

Window guards will prevent the majority of injuries but parents also need to move furniture that children can climb on from under windows, and insist that children do not jump on beds because that often leads to falling out of a nearby window.

Conclusions

Success is increased by a multifaceted approach using product and environment modifications, legislation and enforcement, and public education.

In July 1993, a committee of the National Science Foundation's Institute of Medicine recommended that Congress direct the U.S. Department of Health and Human Services to establish a federal center to conduct, oversee, and coordinate activities related to planning and evaluation, research, and technical assistance in Emergency Medical Services for Children (EMS-C). EMS-C would help combine efforts in prevention, acute care, and rehabilitation. This committee asked that Congress appropriate $30 million annually for five years to support the activities of such a federal center and state agencies responsible for EMS-C.

Emergency Information

Teach Kids How to Use 911

An excellent method for teaching kids how to use the phone to call for help is to make the learning a game. Use a singsong method such as "What do we do when we need help," child answers "911." Most children will not be able to effectively use this information until the age of three, when the child can begin to recognize numbers.

Fire

In case of fire, yell as loud as possible "FIRE!" Do not attempt to put the fire out. Leave the building and do not go back for any reason because although the flames can cause serious injuries it is often the smoke that presents the greatest danger. Therefore, when there is smoke crawl on the floor to the nearest exit and meet at the predetermined family meeting location. Being sure to call the fire department or 911 from a neighbor's home. Also, be certain to teach your children to "stop, drop, and roll."

Earthquake Procedures

The best advice is to be prepared. Evaluate your home and surroundings to ensure that the water heater is braced, anchored, or strapped to prevent tipping and that large furniture is secured to the walls and glass items are stored on lower shelves. Also, make sure that your house is attached to its foundation with bolts. Make sure you have basic emergency supplies including a fire extinguisher, portable radio and extra batteries, flashlights, and enough drinkable water for each family member for three days. Finally, know the safest place in your home and where the shut-offs for the gas, electric, and water main are located.

Develop a family plan that includes an exit for every family member, where to meet, and whom to call out of the area for family notification.

Most importantly, when an earthquake does occur, remain calm and attend to your safety so that if others are injured you are available to provide assistance.

Tornado Procedures

Develop a survival plan for every environment: home, school, and your automobile. Always stay away from windows because of the danger of flying glass. At home or school, try to find the lowest-lying area; this is the safest place to be. If you are in a mobile home—get out; mobile homes are never safe, even when tied down. If you are in a car or a mobile home and adequate shelter is not available, lie in a ditch or on the ground; but be sure to avoid a drainage ditch or storm drain because of the danger of flash floods.

Remember the best advice is to develop an evacuation plan before it is needed and to practice.

What Babysitters, Grandparents, and Caretakers Need to Know

When you are asked to care for children their safety is in your hands [60].

- Have emergency information written down including: family name, children's names, house address with the nearest cross street, instructions on how to contact the parents, phone number(s) of close relatives and neighbors, doctor's name and phone number, the number for the local poison control center, any medication or food allergies, and the children's dates of birth.
- Call 911 or your local emergency number in an emergency.
- Always secure written instructions about medicines, including the correct dose, and when and how to administer the medication.
- Walk through the child's house to familiarize yourself with the surroundings. Know what areas are absolutely off-limits to the children.
- Be sure you know where the children are at all times.

First Aid Basics

Head Trauma

Most important, stay calm; the vast majority of head injuries result in no serious or permanent injury. However, if your child has any of the following symptoms, seek medical attention promptly.

- Bleeding: Scalp wounds bleed dramatically and often seem serious. If the bleeding stops with pressure and there is no deep wound, a clean dressing may be all that is needed. If the bleeding continues despite three to five minutes of gentle pressure, then medical attention should be sought. If the wound is gaping, or bone is visible, medical attention should be sought immediately.
- Loss of consciousness: Even a brief loss of consciousness requires a medical evaluation. Also look for altered consciousness such as amnesia of the event, incoherence, or verbal changes.
- Vomiting: Often with a head injury, the child may vomit once or twice. Nevertheless, if the child vomits more than that he or she needs to be seen by a physician.
- Personality changes: Mild head injuries may produce no obvious symptoms. But following an injury, sometimes over a period of days or weeks, the child's personality may change. This may result from a collection of fluid inside the skull compressing the brain and requires immediate attention by a physician.
- Seizures following a head injury: Seizures following a head injury are not uncommon, but the child should be evaluated as soon as possible.
- Unequal pupils: If pupils are of unequal size by a significant amount the child should be seen by a physician without delay.

Choking

Attempt to remove an object from a child's throat only if you can see it with the mouth open. Otherwise, you might push the object farther down the airway.

If a child is choking but able to breathe and talk, let him or her cough. If not breathing try back blows on an infant or the Heimlich maneuver on older children. Call 911 or your local emergency number immediately.

Poisoning

In your home, have a one-ounce bottle of syrup of ipecac on hand to induce vomiting, but only use when instructed by your pediatrician or the poison control center. The telephone number for the poison control center should be posted near the telephone, and is located in your telephone book. If the child is vomiting, be sure to roll the child on his or her side to avoid choking.

Burns

Burns can be caused by heat (hot water, flames), chemicals, electricity, and the sun. For burns caused by chemicals or electricity, call the local emergency services or 911 immediately. For burns caused by heat, first stop the burning, then apply cool water. Cover the burn with a bandage but do not apply any ointments. Finally, if the burn is severe, noted by whitish or blackened areas, call 911 or your local emergency number immediately and keep the victim from becoming cold through loss of body heat.

Drowning

If a child is removed from water unconscious, CPR should be started immediately and continued until emergency help arrives. If CPR cannot proceed because of a blocked airway, the Heimlich maneuver should be used to dislodge the foreign material, followed by CPR. A second person should call 911 or your local emergency number. Do not stop CPR even if the child remains unresponsive.

Broken Bones

Broken bones require rest, ice, and elevation and are identifiable by extreme pain, twisted limbs, or visible bones. If your child does suffer a broken bone, or you suspect a broken bone, minimize movement. If the break is serious, or you suspect a head or neck injury, do not move the child and call your local emergency services or 911 immediately.

Spinal Cord Injuries

If a child is unconscious, it is important to protect the airway to ensure adequate oxygen is delivered to the brain. In addition, eliminate any movements of the head or torso, which can lead to additional spinal cord damage if there is an unstable injury.

Reference Guide of Resources

Home

United States Consumer Product Safety
  Commission
Washington, DC 20207-0001
1-800-638-2772
www.cpsc.gov

The American Academy of Pediatrics
141 Northwest Point Boulevard
Elk Grove Village, IL 60007-1098
(847) 434-4000
www.aap.org

Children's Safety Network Resource Centers
Children's Safety Network
Education Development Center, Inc.
55 Chapel Street
Newton, MA 02458-1060
(617) 969-7100
www.edc.org

Guide to Baby Products, Fourth Edition
Consumer Reports Books, Sandy Jones
with Werner Freitag and the Editors of
Consumer Reports Books, A Division of
Consumers Union, Yonkers, New York
1994.

The Danny Foundation, Keeping Babies
  Safe
PO Box 680
Alamo, CA 94507
1-800-83DANNY
www.dannyfoundation.org

American Trauma Society
8903 Presidential Parkway
Suite 512
Upper Marlboro, MD 20772
www.amtrauma.org

American Red Cross
431 18th Street, NW
Washington, DC 20006
(202) 639-3520
www.redcross.org

United States Fire Administration (USFA)
Office of Fire Management Programs
16825 South Seton Avenue
Emmitsburg, MD 21727
www.usfa.fema.gov

American Association of Poison Control
  Centers
3201 New Mexico Avenue
Suite 310
Washington, DC 20016
(202) 362-7217
www.aapcc.org

Lead Poisoning Prevention Branch
Division of Environmental Hazards and
  Health Effects
National Center for Environmental Health
1600 Clifton Road, Mailstop E25
Atlanta, GA 30333
(404) 639-2510
www.cdc.gov

Vehicle Safety

National Highway Traffic Safety
    Administration
U.S. DOT/NHTSA, Media and Marketing
    Division, NTS-21
400 7th Street, SW
Washington, DC 20590
(202) 493-2062
Auto Safety Hotline: 1-800-424-9393
Department of Transportation Auto Safety
    Hotline: 1-888-327-4236
www.nhtsa.dot.gov

National SAFE KIDS Campaign
1301 Pennsylvania Avenue, NW
Suite 1000
Washington, DC 20004
(202) 662-0600
www.safekids.org

The Emergency Medical Services for
    Children (EMSC)
111 Michigan Avenue, NW
Washington, DC 20010
(202) 884-4927

AAA Foundation for Traffic Safety
1440 New York Avenue, NW
Suite 201
Washington, DC 20005
(202) 638-5943
www.aafts.org

Playground Safety

National Playground Safety Institute
(703) 820-4940
www.opraonline.org/playgrnd/institut

National Program for Playground Safety
University of Northern Iowa
School for Health, Physical Education, and
    Leisure Services
Cedar Falls, IA 50614-0618
1-800-782-9519
www.uni.edu/playground

United States Consumer Product Safety
    Commission *Handbook for Public Play-
    ground Safety* (Publication Number 325)
Washington, DC 20207-0001
1-800-638-2772
www.cpsc.gov

Pool Safety

Take Cardiopulmonary Resuscitation (CPR)
classes. Classes are offered by both the
American Heart Association and the American Red Cross.

Drowning Prevention Foundation
PO Box 202
Alamo, CA 94507
(925) 820-SAVE
www.drownprevention.com

School Safety

Di Scala, C., Gallagher, S. S., and Schneps,
S. E. (1997). *Journal of School Health,*
67(9): 384–389.

Injuries in the School Environment:
A Resource Guide (2nd Edition) 1997

National Youth Sports Safety
Foundation, Inc.
333 Longwood Avenue
Suite 202
Boston, MA 02115
(617) 277-1171
www.nyssf.org

National Operating Committee on Standards
for Athletic Equipment (NOCSAE)
PO Box 12290
Overland, KS 66282
(913) 888-1340
www.nocsae.org

National Association for the Education
of Young Children
1509 16th Street, NW
Washington, DC 20036-1426
www.naeyc.org

National Association of Child Care
Resource and Referral Agencies
1319 F Street, NW
Suite 810
Washington, DC 20004
1-800-424-2246

Other

National Farm Medicine Center
1000 North Oak Avenue
Marshfield, WI 54449-5790
(715) 389-4999

American Society for Testing and Materials
(ASTM)
100 Barr Harbor Drive
West Conshocken, PA 19428
www.astm.org

BoatU.S. Foundation
880 South Pickett Street
Alexandria, VA 22304
1-800-336-2628
www.boatus.com

National Safe Boating Council, Inc.
PO Box 1058
Delaware, OH 43015-1058
(740) 666-3009
www.safeboatingcouncil.org

United States Coast Guard, Office of Boating
Safety
1-800-368-5647
www.uscgboating.gov

American Heart Association National Center
7272 Greenville Avenue
Dallas, TX 75231
www.americanheart.org

Prevention Strategies

Strategies for Fire and Burn Prevention

- Use only correct size fuses in the fuse box.
- Install and regularly check smoke detectors. Change batteries frequently.
- Teach children to Stop, Drop, and Roll. Be sure to include keeping their faces covered with their hands during the Roll portion.
- Keep a fire extinguisher on hand, know how to use it, and refill it immediately upon use.
- Place and maintain barriers around fireplaces, heaters, radiators, and hot pipes.
- Try not to use matches or lighters around children. If present, store out of sight in a locked cabinet or drawer.
- Teach children to bring you any matches they find. If they find a lighter have them immediately tell you so that you can pick it up.
- Use safety devices to cover electrical outlets.
- Inspect and clean heating systems including stoves and fireplaces once a year.
- Make sure there are sufficient outlets for all appliances to prevent overloading electrical wiring.
- Place smoke alarms around the child care area and check the batteries on a regular basis.
- Keep extension cords exposed; do not run them under furniture or rugs.
- Keep all flammable liquids stored in safety cans and out of reach of children.
- Keep furnaces, heating equipment, and chimneys and flues cleaned regularly.
- Never allow children in food preparation area without supervision.
- Do not drink or carry anything hot when close to a child.
- Test hot food before giving it to a child.

- Never warm a bottle in the microwave.
- Set water heaters to no higher than 120°F.
- Never bathe a child in water you have not tested.
- Never leave children unattended in the bath or near a faucet. They might turn on the hot water.
- Turn pot handles in toward center or rear of stove and only cook on rear burners when possible.
- Never use portable, open-flame, or space heaters.
- Never smoke around children.
- Never store flammable liquids such as gasoline near the child care environment.

Strategies to Prevent Falls Indoors

- Use infant and child equipment that is in good repair and inspected for safety.
- Use durable, balanced furniture that will not tip over easily.
- Do not allow climbing on furniture, stools, or ladders.
- Place safety gates at stairways.
- Remove all objects from stairs.
- Repair or remove frayed carpeting or other flooring.
- Install window guards on upstairs windows.
- Secure all window screens.
- Clean up spills quickly.
- Avoid highly waxed floors and stairways.
- Do not use loose throw rugs.
- Keep toys picked up as often as possible.
- Never leave a baby alone in a high place.

Strategies to Prevent Choking and Suffocation

- Remove loose parts from toys.
- Use a choke testing device on small toys. Always do this before adding a questionable toy to the environment.
- Keep diaper and other pins, toothpicks, and nails out of your mouth.
- Do not wear dangle type jewelry like necklaces and earrings.
- Check toys, games, and art supplies for broken pieces and throw away.
- Teach children not to run with anything in their mouths.
- Teach children to chew well and not allow playing when eating.
- Never prop a baby bottle on the child or bedding.
- Never use Styrofoam cups—children like to chew them.
- Regularly hand out consumer toy alerts as you find them. Newspapers and magazines carry this information, particularly around Christmas.

Outdoor Safety Hazards by Developmental Levels of Age

Age	Hazards	Prevention Tips
0–6 months	Motor Vehicle	Infant should always be in rear-facing infant safety seat and in the backseat.
6 months–1 year	Motor Vehicle	Continue using safety seat; switch to toddler seat when able to sit up by self.
	Poisons	Watch child for mouthing of objects. Check area for poisonous plants.
	Choking	Watch child for mouthing of objects.
	Drowning	Keep pool covered, fenced, and lock gate.
1–2 years	Motor Vehicle	Continue using safety seat.
	Falls	Carefully watch while climbing on outdoor equipment. Teach child safe play practices.
	Equipment	Check playground equipment for rough edges, rust, loose parts. Wood chips or soft sand are best ground coverings under play equipment.
	Poisons	Place all outdoor chemicals, and so forth, in a high place, preferably locked. Check area for poisonous plants.
	Drowning	Cover, fence, and lock gate to pool. Always supervise child when playing near pool or any body of water.
2–3 years	Motor Vehicle	Keep child away from streets and driveways using supervision, fences, and firm discipline. Role model pedestrian behavior such as crossing street. Role model wearing seat belt in car and use safety seat for child.
	Falls	Carefully supervise when on equipment. Reinforce safe behavior on equipment.
	Poisons	Keep poisons up high and locked. Check for poisonous plants.

(continued)

Outdoor Safety Hazards by Developmental Levels of Age (continued)

Age	Hazards	Prevention Tips
2–3 years (continued)	Drowning	Always supervise when near any body of water. Begin to teach water safety, including role modeling. Cover, fence, and lock gate to pool.
	Equipment	Check equipment for hazards. Supervise and role model safety.
3 years and up	Motor Vehicle	Use safety seat or seat belt for child. Teach pedestrian and traffic safety rules. Role model this behavior.
	Equipment	Reinforce safe play habits. Supervise when using tools. Check equipment for hazards.
	Drowning	Children should have swimming lessons if they are in care near a body of water. Teach water safety.
	Violence	Teach children neighborhood safety, including safe houses and familiarity with law enforcement.

Indoor Safety Hazards by Developmental Levels of Age

Age	Hazards	Prevention Tips
6 months–1 year	Choking	Check floors and reachable areas for small objects such as pins, coins, buttons. Avoid raw vegetables, nuts, hard candy, popcorn, and other foods that are difficult for a child to properly chew and swallow.
	Toys	Should be large, unbreakable, and smooth.
	Drowning	Always carefully supervise when bathing.
1–2 years	Falls	Put toddler gates on stairways and keep any doors to cellars, attics, and porches locked. Remove sharp-edged furniture from child's frequently used area. Show child proper way to climb up and down stairs using handrails.

Age	Hazards	Prevention Tips
	Burns	While cooking, turn pot handles to back of stove. Keep electric cords out of reach. Use shock stops to cover used and unused outlets. Teach child the meaning of the word hot and talk about different types of hot.
	Poisons	Keep poisons locked in high cabinets. Have child tested for lead poisoning during regular check-up.
	Drowning	Always supervise child's bath.
	Choking	Remove small objects.
2–3 years	Poisons	Teach child about the difference between food and non-food and what is not good to eat. Watch child during art projects so he does not put art supplies in mouth. Keep poisons locked in high cabinets.
	Burns	Keep matches, lighter, and cigarettes out of reach and sight of children. Put screen around fireplaces and wood stoves. Reinforce the meaning of "hot."
	Toys	Check for sharp edges, hinges, and small parts that could be swallowed. Remove toy chest lids.
	Drowning	Always supervise.
	Guns	Keep any firearms unloaded and locked away out of reach.
3 years and up	Burns	Teach child drop and roll to prepare for clothing catching fire. Practice fire drills with escape route meeting place and sound of smoke alarm. Train to bring found matches to adult.
	Tools and equipment	Teach child safe use of scissors. Keep sharp knives out of reach.
	Guns	Keep firearms unloaded and locked. Teach safety precautions about guns, instructing children to tell an adult immediately when they see a gun and not to touch it. Discourage use of toy guns or violent play.

(From *Safety, Nutrition and Health in Early Education*, by Cathie Robertson, Delmar/Thomson Learning © 1998)

bibliography

1. Stylianos, S., & Eichelberger, M. R. (1993). Pediatric trauma: Prevention strategies. *Pediatric Clinics of North America*, 40, 1359–1368.

2. Cooper, A., & Barlow, B. (1995) The surgeon and emergency medical services for children. *Pediatrics, 96*, 184–188.

3. Moront, M. L., Williams, J. A., Eichelberger, M. R., et al. (1994). The injured child: An approach to care. *Pediatric Clinics of North America, 41*, 1201–1226.

4. Stylianos, S. (1992). Pediatric trauma: The injured family. In B. H. Harris and J. L. Grosfeld (Eds.), *Progress in pediatric trauma* (4th ed., pp. 76E–76I). Boston: Nobb Hill.

5. Lisa Carter and Lori Marques. (2000, May 29). www.paranoidsisters.com.

6. American Academy of Pediatrics. (2000, May 29). *Family shopping guide to car seats.* www.aap.org/family/famshop.html.

7. Sosin, et al. (1996). *Pediatrics, 11*, 868–870.

8. U.S. Department of Transportation. (1998). *Annual report.* Washington, DC: U.S. Department of Transportation.

9. National Program for Playground Safety, Mack, M. G., Hudson, S., & Thompson, D. (1997). A descriptive analysis of children's playground injuries in the United States, 1990–94. *Injury Prevention, 3*, 100–103.

10. Centers for Disease Control and Prevention. (1997).

11. National Program for Playground Safety, University of Northern Iowa, Cedar Falls, IA. 1-800–5554–PLAY.

12. National Safekids. (2000, March). Gun Safety Initiative, Press Release. www.safekids.org.

13. Wade, S., Taylor, H.G., Drotar, D., Stancin, T., & Yeates, K. O. (1996). Childhood traumatic brain injury: Initial impact on the family. *Journal of Learning Disabilities, 26*(6), 658.

14. Meyer, E. C., Snelling, L. K., & Myren-Manbeck, L. (1998). Pediatric intensive care: The parents' experience. *Clinical Issues, 9*(1), 69.

15. Conoley, J. C., & Sheridan, S. M. (1996). Pediatric traumatic brain injury: Challenges and interventions for families. *Journal of Learning Disabilities, 29*(6), 663–664.

16. Breslau, N., & Prabucki, K. (1987). Siblings of disabled children: Effects of chronic stress in the family. *Archives of General Psychiatry, 44*, 1042–1044.

17. Bullock, M. (1981). The grief-relief process: Coping with the life and death of physically and mentally disabled children. *Orthopedic Clinic of North America, 12*(1), 197.

18. Wesson, et al.

19. Lynch, M. L. *Creating an optimal rehabilitation environment: A cooperative effort.*

20. Breslau, N., Staruch, K. S., & Mortimer, E. A. (1982). Psychological distress in mothers of disabled children. *American Journal for Diseases of Children, 136,* 682–685.

21. Bronan, & Michel (Eds.). (1995). Traumatic head injury in children. In *Recovery from traumatic brain injury in children: The importance of the family.* Oxford.

22. Molner, G. E. (Ed.). (1995). *Pediatric rehabilitation.* Philadelphia: Williams & Wilkins.

23. Baumer, J. H., Wadsworth, J., & Taylor, B. (1988). Family recovery after death of a child. *Archives of Disease in Childhood, 63,* 946.

24. Van Eijk, J. Smits, A., Huygen, F., & Van Den Hoogen, V. (1988). Effect of bereavement on the health of the remaining family members. *Family Practice, 5*(4), 281.

25. Sanders, C. M. (1979–1980). A Comparison of adult bereavement in the death of a spouse, child and parent. *Omega, 10*(4), 310.

26. Cowan, M. E., & Murphy, S. A. (1985). Identification of Postdisaster Bereavement Risk Predictors. *Nursing Research, 34*(2), 77.

27. Back, K. J. (1991). Sudden, unexpected pediatric death: Caring for the parents. *Pediatric Nursing, 17*(6), 572.

28. Schaefer, D., & Lyons, C. (1993). *How do we tell the children? A step-by-step guide for helping children two to teens cope when someone dies.* New York: Newmarket Press.

29. Parrott, C. (1992). *Parents' grief: Help and understanding after the death of a baby.* Washington, DC: Medic Publishing Co.

30. Bell, J. & Esterling, L. S. (1986). *What will I tell the children?* University of Nebraska

Medical Center Child Life Department and Munroe-Meyer Institution.

31. NFO Research, Inc. on behalf of Compassionate Friends. (1999, June). *When a child dies: A survey of bereaved parents.*

32. Agran, P., Winn, D., & Dunkle, D. (1989). Injuries among 4–9 year old restrained motor vehicle occupants by seat location and crash impact site. *American Journal of Diseases of Children, 143,* 1317–1321.

33. Barlow, B., Niemerska, M., Gandhi, R. P., et al. (1983). Ten years of experience with falls from a height in children. *Journal of Pediatric Surgery, 18,* 509–511.

34. Bergman, A. B., Rivara, F. P., Richards, D. D., et al. (1990). The Seattle children's bicycle helmet campaign. *American Journal of Diseases of Children, 144,* 727–731.

35. Bjornstig, U., Ostrom, M., Eriksson, A., et al. (1992). Head and face injuries in bicyclists with special reference to possible effects of helmet use. *Journal of Trauma, 33,* 887–893.

36. Bull, M. J., Stroup, K. B., Gerhart, S. (1988). Misuse of car safety seats. *Pediatrics, 81,* 98–101.

37. Cooper, A., Barlow, B., Davidson, L. L., et al. (1990). Epidemiology of pediatric trauma: Importance of population based data. *Journal of Pediatric Surgery, 27,* 1–6.

38. Davidson, L. L., Durkin, M. S., O'Connor, P., et al. (1992). The epidemiology of severe injuries to children in northern Manhattan: Methods and incidence rates. *Pediatric Perinatal Epidemiology, 6,* 153–165.

39. DiGuiseppi, C. G., Rivara, F. P., Koepsell, T. D., et al. (1989). Bicycle helmet use by children: Evaluation of a community-wide helmet campaign. *Journal of the American Medical Association, 262,* 2256–2261.

40. Gorman, R. L., Charfney, E., Holtzman, N. A., et al. (1985). A successful city-wide smoke detector giveaway program. *Pediatrics, 75*, 14–18.

41. Gotschall, C. S. (1992). Epidemiology of childhood injury. In M. R. Eichelberger (Ed.), *Pediatric trauma: Prevention, acute care, and rehabilitation* (pp. 16–19). St. Louis: Mosby-Yearbook.

42. Gotschall, C. S., Mickalide, A. D., & Eichelberger, M. R. (1992). Childhood injury prevention and control. In R. Dieckmann (Ed.), *Pediatric emergency care systems* (pp. 91–100). Philadelphia: Williams and Wilkins.

43. Haddon, W. (1968). The changing approach to the epidemiology, prevention, and amelioration of trauma. *American Journal of Public Health, 58*, 1431–1438.

44. Haddon, W. (1973). Energy damage and the ten countermeasure strategies. *Journal of Trauma, 13*, 321.

45. Harris, B. H., Latchaw, L. A., Murphy, R. E., et al. (1989). A protocol for pediatric trauma receiving units. *Journal of Pediatric Surgery, 24*, 419–422.

46. Jumbelic, M. I., & Chambliss, M. (1990). Accidental toddler drowning in 5-gallon buckets. *Journal of the American Medical Association, 263*, 1952–1953.

47. Maull, K. I. (1989). Dispelling fatalism in a cause and effect world. *Journal of Trauma, 29*, 752–756.

48. Miller, R. E., Reisinger, K. S., Blatter, M. M., et al. (1982). Pediatric counseling and subsequent use of smoke detectors. *American Journal of Public Health, 72*, 392–393.

49. Newman, K. D., Bowman, L. M., Eichelberger, M. R., et al. (1990). The lap belt complex: Intestinal and lumbar spine injury in children. *Journal of Trauma, 30*, 1133–1140.

50. Pearn, J., & Nixon, J. (1977). Prevention of childhood drowning accidents. *Medical Journal of Aust., 1*, 616–618.

51. Rivara, F. P. (1992). Control of childhood injury. In M. R. Eichelberger (Ed.), *Pediatric trauma: Prevention, acute care, and rehabilitation* (pp. 11–15). St Louis: Mosby-Yearbook.

52. Rivara, F. P. (1990). Child pedestrian injuries in the United States. *American Journal of Diseases of Children, 144*, 692–696.

53. Spence, L. J., Dykes, E. H., Bohn, D. J., et al. (1993). Fatal bicycle accidents in children: A plea for prevention. *Journal of Pediatric Surgery, 28*, 214–216.

54. Stylianos, S., & Harris, B. H. (1990). Seatbelt use and patterns of central nervous system injury in children. *Pediatric Emergency Care, 6*, 4–5.

55. Thompson, R. S., Rivara, F. P., & Thompson, D. C. (1989). A case-control study of the effectiveness of bicycle safety helmets. *New England Journal of Medicine, 320*, 1361–1367.

56. Walton, W. (1982). An evaluation of the Poison Packaging Prevention Act. *Pediatrics, 69*, 363–370.

57. Wintemute, G. J. (1990). Childhood drowning and near-drowning in the United States. *American Journal of Diseases of Children, 144*, 663–669.

58. Centers for Disease Control and Prevention. (1985). Update: Childhood poisonings—United States. *Morbidity and Mortality Weekly Report, 34*, 26–27.

59. Division of Injury Control, Centers for Disease Control and Prevention. (1990). Childhood injuries in the United States. *American Journal of Diseases of Children, 144*, 627–646.

60. Los Angeles City Fire Department, Captain Bud Gundersen. (2000, May 29). Children's Safety Zone Home Page. www.sosnet.com.